ALSO BY JOHN W. FARQUHAR, M.D.

The American Way of Life Need Not Be
Hazardous to Your Health

THE
LAST
PUFF

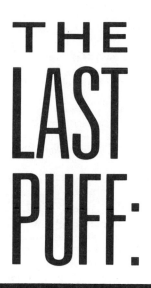

THE
LAST
PUFF:

EX-SMOKERS SHARE THE
SECRETS OF THEIR SUCCESS

JOHN W. FARQUHAR, M.D.
GENE A. SPILLER, PH.D.

W. W. NORTON & COMPANY
NEW YORK LONDON

Printed in the United States of America.

The text of this book is composed in 11/15 Baskerville, with display type set in Univers 49 and 63. Composition and manufacturing by The Haddon Craftsmen, Inc. Book design by Jo Anne Metsch.

First published as a Norton paperback 1991

Library of Congress Cataloging-in-Publication Data

Farquhar, John W.
The last puff: ex-smokers share the secrets of their success
John W. Farquhar, Gene A. Spiller.—1st ed.
p.   cm.
1. Ex-smokers—Interviews.   2. Cigarette smokers—Psychology—Case
studies.   3. Tobacco habit.   I. Spiller, Gene A.   II. Title.
HV5748.F37 1990
613.85—dc20   89–16182

ISBN 0-393-30803-0

W. W. Norton & Company, Inc., 500 Fifth Avenue, New York, N.Y. 10110
W. W. Norton & Company Ltd, 10 Coptic Street, London WC1A 1PU

0

For C. Everett Koop, who as Surgeon General of the United States courageously worked for a smoke-free country.

And for the ex-smokers whose stories and ideas made this book possible.

CONTENTS

CONTENTS

AUTHORS' NOTE

The idea for this book came to us when we realized that there was no popular book in which ex-smokers tell their own stories of how they were successful in giving up the habit. We already knew that the great majority of people who have quit—approximately 95 percent, according to recent research—have done so on their own. How did they do it? we wondered. What made them successful—finally? We decided to interview men and women of all ages and many different professions, to try and answer these questions.

The interviews (Chapter 4) are the heart of the book. In the ex-smokers' own words, they reflect their inner feelings and reveal how each person stopped in his or her own way, often inventing a special method. Chapters 1, 2, and 3 set the stage for the stories, and Chapters 5, 6, and 7 discuss some of the highlights of these stories in view of our current knowledge of smoking and addiction.

We want to express our thanks to our many colleagues at the Stanford Center for Research in Disease Prevention, who have contributed so much to our thinking about the issues of smoking and health and whose research is of inestimable help in the battle against nicotine addiction.

A special acknowledgment goes to Christine Farquhar, for her valuable writing and editing skills as *The Last Puff* developed; to Carol Kino, who aided in designing and setting up the early interviews; to Margaret Denny, for her editorial assistance; to Sara Godwin, who carried out some of the interviews and was very valuable in the final stages of manuscript preparation; and to Becki Carr, who transcribed many hours of taped interviews with great professional skill.

A special role was played by Carol Houck Smith of W. W. Norton. From the inception of this work to final edited manuscript, this book would not have been possible without her deep involvement. Her skillful editing and her many suggestions have made this book what it is now. As an ex-smoker as well as an editor, she brought her personal feelings and knowledge to the book in a unique way.

THE
LAST
PUFF

DIFFERENT KEYS,
DIFFERENT LOCKS

What is the pivotal event that makes it possible for someone to quit smoking permanently, often after a long period of excruciating failures? Why do some people decide to give up the habit and never touch another
cigarette, while others fail miserably in their repeated
attempts to quit smoking?

Consider for example the story of Dick W., a fifty-
nine-year-old man. He is a smoker now, but he has tried
to quit many times. Once he was successful for fifteen
years!

"I had smoked for about eighteen years, from 1948 to
1966, when four of us at work had the urge to quit
smoking: We each took $500 and gave it to a fifth person
to hold. Anybody who smoked during the course of a
year would lose his interest in the pot, and anybody who

held out to the end would split the pot.

"Of the three other guys who quit with me, one started to smoke again within two months, another one within six months, so the third guy and I split the $2,000 pot.

"I made it through the next fourteen years without a cigarette, but in 1980 my wife died very, very suddenly. She was only forty-eight and she died in her sleep one night—probably of diabetes.

"I had a cigarette within twenty-four hours after she died. Somebody offered me a cigarette, and I've wanted to cuss him out ever since. I smoked one, and that one led to another, and another led to another. All I had to do was touch one.

"It was the trauma of my wife dying, the sorrow.

"I know I shouldn't be smoking, but I married again at the end of 1982. My new wife is a very heavy smoker, and it's extremely difficult to have just one partner in a marriage give up cigarettes. About a year after we were married we made a pact that we would quit, and we did quit for a month or two. But she was having trouble with her teen-age son and she went back to smoking. That made it very easy for me to go back too. We quit again the first of this year for about a month. I don't know why we started smoking again.

"We keep talking about quitting again. We both want to quit."

While many people will find Dick W.'s story all too familiar, many others have succeeded in conquering their addiction to smoking. It is fascinating to unravel the mysteries of quitting to see how a person evolves from being a smoker to being a non-smoker. The best way to observe the process is to let former smokers tell us why and how they quit.

That is what this book is all about. It's a collection of real, intriguing life stories of people who have successfully quit smoking. You'll meet people from all walks of life, men and women of all ages. You may identify more with some of these people than others, but you should read all the stories. Every one contains fascinating insights into the goals, failures, and ultimate triumph of a former smoker. And each carries the message of hope: You *can* quit smoking. All of these people have done it.

There are about 43 million adult Americans who have given up smoking since 1967. Until now, no one has officially asked them how they did it or gathered their stories in a book. Ninety-five percent or so of those 43 million quit without the help of formal clinics or classes. They quit on their own, by themselves. They did it their own way, every one a different approach, every one a successful solution.

Can the interviews in this book help the 65 million people in the United States who still smoke? Ninety-five percent of those who would like to stop will do it by marshaling their own resources, as most people do. When people see their own experience in someone else's story, they often know better what to do and how to do it and can even gain the courage to do it.

THE FIRST SUCCESS STORY:
SOMETHING CLICKED

Fortunately, ex-smokers are willing to share the secrets of their success. Of course, they deserve to have pride in their accomplishments, but we've also found that people respond in a marvelous way to the idea of helping their fellow humans. That's the spirit you'll find in this book.

For the moment now, John Farquhar is not the physician, the cardiologist involved in preventive medicine who is one of the authors of this book. Instead, John is an ex-smoker, relaxing on his sofa at home and telling his own story. The tape recorder is running. . . .

"When I graduated from high school it was wartime, and I was recruited into a college program called the Army Specialized Training Reserve program. I was seventeen. Toward the end of my first year, I met a girl from California. She was a smoker. We danced to the recordings of the Glenn Miller band and we fell in love. She taught me to smoke. Smoking seemed very sophisticated and very much the right thing to do for a young man in love in wartime. Three months later I was shipped out to basic training. I quit smoking for several months, but the Army's weekly ration of free cigarettes got me started again, and I smoked my way through most of the Occupation.

"In Europe I quit for a while for economic reasons. Our post in Belgium was responsible for shipping the

American troops home. It was standard operating procedure for returning American soldiers to deal in the black market. The opportunity to exchange those free cigarettes for cameras and things of that sort was a very strong motivation to stop smoking. I stayed off cigarettes while I was in Belgium in 1946, and in Germany later on, as well.

"By the time I returned to the United States at age nineteen, I had already started and stopped smoking several times. I started smoking again as an undergraduate at UCLA. I was in a fraternity, and I think the percentage of men who smoked was well over 75 percent. In the immediate postwar era it was standard for men to smoke, particularly those who had been through World War II in any way, shape, or form. I was a confirmed smoker throughout college, four years of medical school, one year of internship, and three and a half years of residency. I was a pack-a-day smoker, as most people were.

"I particularly recall smoking during my internship and residency. There is a certain set formality to making ward rounds in a hospital. It's done in the morning, we were expected to be there fairly early, and we were expected to see every patient. There would be an intern, a medical student, a couple of residents, and perhaps the chief resident, all making the rounds together. We always had an aluminum cart on wheels, about five feet high and three and a half feet wide, which held two rows of patients' charts with aluminum covers on them and a patient's name on each of the slots in front.

"Well, on the top of that chart cart we'd have a couple

19

of ashtrays. Perhaps one out of four or five of us didn't smoke, but by and large, everyone smoked. We would have our cigarettes in our mouths outside in the hall and we would be smoking and taking a puff and talking about the case and then we would go into the room. If it was a one-bed room or a two-bed room, we would tend to leave our cigarettes burning on the ashtray outside and go in and come out before the cigarette had burned up. But if it was a four-bed room or a six-bed room, we would wheel the cart in and we would go to the bedside. We didn't keep the cigarettes in our mouths while we were listening through the stethoscope—we had enough politeness and wisdom to leave the smoking cigarettes in the ashtray at least—but that's what we did.

"The patients were often very sick, maybe they even had major lung disease, but no one considered whether or not it might be bad for them to have four or five people smoking in their room. It never even occurred to us that it might smell bad, or leave a lingering stale tobacco odor, or offend someone. Why would we consider esthetics when we didn't have the awareness, as physicians, to consider the impact on our patients' health? The whole attitude of society toward smoking was completely different then. We were men; men smoked.

"And there were cigarette machines in the hospital lobby. The patients were smoking, so you would have these hospital rooms full of smoke. That was just the norm.

"There was absolutely no pressure on us in medical school not to smoke. And by this time I had finished my residency and I had finished a year and a half of a post-doctoral fellowship in cardiology, so I was a fully trained physician.

"The only pressure came from my father, who kept after me in a subtle but persistent way. He had been an athlete when he was younger, and he knew instinctively that smoking was bad for the body, but when he would say I should stop he found it difficult to explain why. He just said that it wasn't good for me, and then I'd say, under my breath, 'Well, *I'm* the doctor. What do *you* know?' I dismissed his instinctive knowledge.

"But thinking about the origin of his opposition to smoking, I remember a story he told me about his father, an immigrant from Scotland who lived in Canada. He and his wife raised a large family—there were thirteen children and eight survivors—and his father was a very religious man. Once he caught one of my father's brothers, David, out in the barn smoking. And he said, 'If the good Lord had intended you to smoke, He would have put a smokestack up on the top of your head.' I am guessing that my father may have absorbed a kind of ethos from his father about smoking being wrong.

"In 1958 I had completed my training and was getting ready to move to New York City to work at the Rockefeller Institute for Medical Research. I developed bronchitis. I was coughing, and I knew I had to leave for New York in about a week. It was about eight o'clock at night and I was in a little, damp, musty, windowless San Francisco basement study. I was sitting at my desk and very intense about getting things done that I had to get done.

I remember to this day how I felt. I had been sick. I had a bad cold and it had stayed in my lungs; I had bronchitis, and I kept coughing. I was smoking at my desk as usual and I took a deep puff. I inhaled it, blew it out the way you do in ordinary smoking, and as I did, I coughed. I can remember, I had the cigarette in my hand, and I coughed. Suddenly something clicked. I said to myself, 'Hey, this is crazy. Here you are, you've got bronchitis, you breathe in the cigarette smoke, and it makes you cough. That's dumb.' At that moment I quit.

"I had no plans to quit. I had never even thought about quitting before. I hadn't written down a quit date, I hadn't read anything about how you're supposed to do it, and I didn't know anyone who had quit. But from that night on, I have never had a cigarette. After I stopped, I think I probably got a little stubborn about staying off. But there was a weird thing: There were people in my life who were very close to me who knew I smoked. I chose not to announce the fact that I'd quit, and for two weeks no one noticed that I'd stopped smoking. I was upset. Here I'd done something difficult and I was proud of myself and nobody even noticed.

"Did I suffer? I did. I remember being irritable. I remember a good deal of irritability, stress, and discomfort, but I got through by invoking a spirit of stubbornness within. I gave myself a very strong message: 'You are now a non-smoker and you are not going to smoke any more.' Within a few months, I didn't have any desire to smoke.

"Eventually I became the kind of person that a lot of

ex-smokers are. You become very, very aware of other people's smoking. I can sniff it out and don't like it at all. Some of my friends tell me that they'll have a nightmare and imagine they are going back, but I don't remember any of that. I don't remember dreams, and I don't remember feeling tempted.

"I've told the medical students in a course I teach in personal health that I wish I'd had teachers who said something about what was good for *our* health. In the first year of medical school there was one doctor who said we ought to have good posture, and he tried to show us what good posture was. Beyond that, it was straight science. We weren't taught how to take care of ourselves; we were taught how to treat various diseases. There was not one whisper about, 'You ought to take care of yourself, you ought to get enough sleep, you ought to eat sensibly, you ought to exercise, you ought to maintain a reasonable weight.' Certainly, no one ever said you shouldn't smoke." The tape recorder is off, John's interview is over.

FORM A BOND WITH SUCCESS

Imagine the interviews in this book as a lock and key. Each lock-and-key combination opens the doors to different houses or cars, but the result is the same: They let you into your own house or car. The diversity in quitting methods is like different keys opening different locks, but the result—quitting—is the same. There is a different lock and a different key for each individual.

What you need to do, then, is find the key among the stories in this book that opens *your* own door to quitting successfully. Look at each key and decide whether it will work for you. The more you see of yourself in the story of someone who used a particular key, the better that key will fit you.

In smoking cessation classes, the participants' smoking histories are revealed and shared by the whole group before they move on to quitting techniques. The problems that each individual encounters on the way toward non-smoking are shared as well. The class develops a group spirit. There is camaraderie, a spirit of helping that extends beyond quitting smoking.

That same spirit of helping and sharing is present in the interviews that follow. If you are a smoker, be inspired, get motivated, learn from these people. They can teach you the tricks of the trade, things that we in medicine don't necessarily have in our bag of tricks. In the interviews you'll hear your own voice coming back to you.

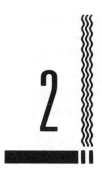

THE LIFE OF A SMOKER: FROM FIRST TO LAST PUFF

Each smoker's story is different, fascinating, and unique, from the first cigarette to the very last. However, as individual as these stories are, as different as the individual lives may be, they have in common some typical developmental events:

1. The difficult, often nauseating first puff
2. The social pressure to smoke
3. The addiction, physical and psychological
4. A period of heavy smoking with no thought of quitting
5. An incubation period of attempts to quit and relapses
6. A triggering event that leads to quitting (often with a device or personal gimmick)

7. A phase of missing cigarettes and loving secondhand smoke
8. The final phase, when the ex-smoker rejects smoking and typically objects to others who smoke

THE LEARNING PROCESS

The interesting thing about smoking is that it's actually very difficult to get started because the initial experience is usually unpleasant. That first puff can be pretty vile, and many people who never became smokers say it's because they couldn't stand the taste of the first cigarette, so they never had another. One puff is often all it takes to make novice smokers dizzy or nauseated. Inhaling is enough to bring tears to their eyes and make them cough. Lots of first-time smokers feel themselves turning green and end up throwing up. Young people who experiment with smoking sometimes play tough and hide from their friends that they think it's awful. The real wonder is that anybody manages to get through the *first puff* to become addicted to nicotine.

Even though it usually takes a long time before inhaling can be carried off gracefully, new smokers pick up the social aspects of smoking very quickly. We sometimes refer to this as the *acculturation* process. People learn when to light up and when not to. They imitate the style of smokers they admire, in hopes of appearing more mature and in control. By careful observation they learn how to hold the cigarette properly, how to inhale without coughing wildly, and how to affect an appropriately sophisticated expression to go with their newly acquired savoir-faire.

Many people go through the process of learning to smoke secretly and in private, wondering why they are doing it, until the unanticipated moment when the nicotine itself begins to take hold and causes a physical addiction. By then, they may already be psychologically addicted. It takes from six months to a year to get hooked on nicotine.

ADDICTION

Being hooked is another way of saying *addicted.* It's ironic: The smoker who may well have had a tough time getting used to smoking now cannot get through a day without cigarettes. Deprived of the opportunity to smoke for a few hours, the serious smoker will fantasize about smoking, feel desperately uncomfortable, become twitchy and nervous, and go to great lengths to get a cigarette.

Some smokers go out at three in the morning and drive through snow to get a pack of cigarettes. Others pay a small fortune for theater tickets and then run out to the lobby every thirty minutes for a cigarette break, missing a third of the play in the process. This is addiction; this is being hooked on tobacco. Sounds familiar, doesn't it? And yet now people talk about nicotine addiction as if it were a brand-new discovery!

Morphine, cocaine, and nicotine have these features in common:

They are all drugs that act on the brain and the nerves, such as the nerves in the spinal cord.

The spread of dependence is socially mediated and is persistent; relapse is common.

Use persists in the face of serious damage, both individual and social.

These drugs are *psychoactive euphoriants,* two big words that really mean they make you feel happy. Tolerance and physical dependence are produced by repeated drug administration. Tolerance means that after a person has used the drug for a while it takes a bigger dose to produce the same "feel-good" effect. In the case of nicotine, the smoker goes from a couple of cigarettes a day to a pack a day or more.

It is possible, and even likely, that some people are more susceptible to nicotine addiction than others. It is clear that the addiction to nicotine is as strong as the addiction to heroin. The evidence for the powerful hold of nicotine is frightening. If you take people who are smokers and withhold cigarettes from them but give them syringes containing nicotine, they will inject nicotine into their veins, exactly like heroin addicts.

Psychological Addiction

Psychological addiction is closely interwoven with lifestyle. All smokers develop their own habits of smoking: while drinking coffee, talking on the telephone, or driving the car, or after sex. Stress often triggers the urge: having a quarrel, getting caught in traffic, hearing upsetting news. Pleasant situations such as chatting at a party, having a drink with friends, or relaxing after dinner also trigger the desire for a cigarette. Sometimes the trigger is no more than wanting to have something to do with your hands or the familiar ritual of lighting up.

The Russian physiologist Pavlov, in famous experiments with dogs, showed that if a bell was rung whenever the dog was fed, after a few weeks the bell alone would cause the dog to salivate, even if there wasn't any food. Smokers become conditioned in a similar way. They smoke in the context of their daily activities, and after a while certain activities associated with smoking become in themselves a stimulus to smoke.

In the smoking narratives in Chapter 4 you'll read about people who, after stopping smoking, began to play with pens and pencils to keep their hands busy, or ate candy and chewed gum to deal with their desire for oral gratification. They still felt the stimulus to smoke, but they substituted other activities for smoking.

Physical Addiction

Physical addiction is less understood, and much of what is known has been withheld from the American public. This information needs to be made public and emphasized to help young people choose not to smoke.

There are centers in the brain that are crucial in transmitting nervous impulses. These centers use specific chemical substances—*neurotransmitters*—that are synthesized at the end of the nerve, ready to transfer impulses to the next nerve cells. These *nerve endings* become saturated with nicotine, which acts as a substitute neurotransmitter that produces a "jolt" in the brain. The brain records nicotine in these nerve cells as the psychological feelings of tranquility and alertness, and that leads to *dependency* or *physical addiction.*

Research may provide ways to prevent nicotine from affecting the transmission of signals in the brain. For now, the best way to prevent addiction is not to smoke.

The key feature of addiction is that if you do not have the drug, you crave it. And after you take the addicting substance regularly for a long period of time, you become so used to it that you slowly find you need more and more of the substance to get the same effect. This is what happens with nicotine.

Another feature of addiction is that you continue doing it even though it doesn't taste good or feel good and you know it's bad for you. Studies of committed smokers—those famous pack-a-day "average" smokers—have shown that the smoker *wants* only three or four cigarettes a day. The others are smoked to keep the blood level of nicotine up, that is, to satisfy the physical addiction. Watch the faces of addicted smokers having their first puff after not smoking for two or three hours. They will draw the smoke in deeply, hold it a long time, and let it out slowly. A wave of relaxation and pleasure spreads over their faces. That is the nicotine fix.

The most frightening aspect of nicotine addiction is that people will continue their dangerous behavior despite known harm to their health and their bodies, and even when they have personally experienced the consequences they continue to smoke. Some people who have emphysema or who have had a cancerous lung removed continue to smoke in spite of the devastating damage they have suffered. That demonstrates the terrible strength of the addiction to nicotine.

Serious smokers know exactly how many cigarettes to smoke, and when, in order to keep their nicotine level up so they don't start to feel bad. The brain signals, "Okay, it's time," and the smoker starts checking pockets or purse for the pack of cigarettes. Before smokers get on a two-hour flight on an airline where smoking is banned, they are likely to take a few extra-deep puffs because they know the fix has to last. Nicotine produces effects that are considered therapeutic by users; that's part of the euphoriant, "feel-good" effect.

It's important to recognize the connection between nicotine addiction and heroin addiction: The curve of relapse for people who have quit taking heroin and that for people who have stopped smoking are almost identical. In less technical language, nicotine is as addictive as heroin, and the habit is as hard to kick. It is shocking to contemplate that in the United States it is legal to produce, advertise, and sell a drug that is so dangerous to health and so addictive. It seriously threatens the health of the smoker as well as the health of those who merely breathe the cigarette smoke. No government in the world would allow that for heroin!

When cigarette labels were changed a few years ago,

the government did order the cigarette companies to label cigarettes with a variety of warnings about the dangers of low birthweight, heart disease, and various cancers and the fact that nicotine is addictive. The end result was a political compromise. The tobacco industry agreed to include all the health warnings on the warning labels as long as they did not have to state that nicotine is addictive. There is not a cigarette package in the United States that warns smokers that if they use the product exactly as it is intended to be used they will become addicted to a deadly poison—but that is, in fact, the case.

SHARED ADDICTIONS

People who are addicted to one drug often experiment with other drugs, and multiple addictions are not uncommon. Addiction to nicotine, either physical or psychological, is often combined with addiction to other psychoactive drugs, such as alcohol. Studies have shown that the rate of cigarette addiction in adult alcoholics is as high as 90 percent; it is almost universal that people who drink heavily also smoke heavily.

There is more to consider about the mixture of nicotine and alcohol: People who use alcohol increase the number of cigarettes they smoke as they increase the amount of alcohol they drink. In addition, the way they smoke a cigarette changes. Studies show that drinkers inhale more often and more deeply while drinking. Heavy drinkers who smoke inhale the carcinogenic substances of tobacco more deeply than non-drinkers do. This may explain why cancers of the mouth, pharynx, and esophagus are more common in people who drink and smoke: Not only do they tend to smoke more cigarettes, but they inhale more deeply as well.

People hooked on cigarettes to this extent generally do not entertain serious thoughts of quitting.

THE INCUBATION PERIOD: WEIGHING THE PROS AND CONS

Needless to say, the essential first step in quitting is the decision to stop smoking. Most people consider this step carefully, thinking about it for weeks, months, even years. But they usually don't succeed in their first attempt, which may last only a few hours or days. What's important is that for most people there is an *incubation period,* a time of mulling it over, weighing the pros and cons, that precedes the attempt to quit.

Since 1964, the knowledge of the dangers of cigarettes has made the incubation period more active, because people have become increasingly uncomfortable with smoking. Even when they deny it, they have a nagging suspicion that they shouldn't be smoking. Active incubation includes reading, listening, thinking, analyzing, mulling, denying, questioning, and gathering information. It's one step on the road to motivation.

Failed Attempts and Relapses

As Mark Twain observed, "Quitting smoking is easy; I've done it a thousand times." Many people stop smoking briefly and then suffer a relapse. While Mark Twain's "thousand times" may be an exaggeration for most people—four or five is the norm—a relapse should not send you back to the dungeon. Most people return to the active incubation period, gather more information, marshal more courage and more resolve, and make another serious quitting attempt.

The causes of relapse in smokers have mystified researchers, because after about two weeks all traces of nicotine are gone from the body. Why then is relapse so common?

The two most common reasons are paradoxical: Relapse can occur when the person is in a pleasant, happy situation, or when he is unhappy or under unusual stress. In happy circumstances, such as social situations where alcohol and food are present and other people are smoking, the warm friendliness of the atmosphere sweeps the new ex-smoker back into smoking. That slip of resolve can make the ex-smoker lose faith in her willpower, say "What the hell," and start smoking again. After a week or so, the smoker is not only physically addicted again but disappointed and discouraged about the ability to ever quit once and for all.

The stress factor, our second reason for relapse, is intriguing. Many people who are fired, move from one part of the country to another, go through a divorce, have a serious illness in the family, or experience problems at work start smoking again impulsively. They remember smoking as a stress reliever. There appears to be some sort of residual memory in the nervous system that remains imprinted long after all traces of nicotine have disappeared from the body. What is left that is so indelibly printed on the psychic memory? At this point, science has no answer.

THE TRIGGERING EVENT

After all this incubation, sensitizing, relapsing, something happens—major or minor—that triggers the final attempt at the last puff.

The death of a close friend or member of the family, a personal illness, or some sort of social pressure may make the smoker more sensitive to his smoking habit. These sensitizing episodes can be something major, like a death, or very minor, like being asked to smoke outside a building or not to smoke in somebody's house. Smokers become more acutely aware of a personal habit and are likely to consider the personal and social ramifications every time they light up. Smoking then changes from an unthinking act, an unconscious habit, to a conscious choice each time the smoker takes out a cigarette.

The trigger may be internal or external, in the form of incentives or pressures from without. People are quite ingenious about the incentive, gimmick, or method they use to stop. This rich experience in quitting methods is, perhaps, the heart of this book. Whether it comes from without or within, the trigger is what leads to finally quitting, once and for all.

MISSING CIGARETTES

During the first few weeks, and sometimes for as long as the first few months, ex-smokers have sudden, unexpected urges to smoke. The brain, with all its complex connections and the many chemicals it produces to transmit signals from one nerve cell to another, has become dependent on nicotine. Since nicotine is both a tranquilizer and a stimulant, the brain misses both the calming, relaxing effect and the stimulating effect. When deprived of nicotine, those cells say, "Where is it? Where is it? I want it. I want it." Eventually, as the toxins are diminished in the body, the cells adjust to doing without nicotine, and the craving becomes less frequent and less intense, although sometimes the memory of cigarette smoking as a tranquilizer and stimulant leaves the brain thinking that maybe it ought to go back to it, even after the physiological addiction is gone.

After a few weeks the body is back to normal, however, and is no longer physically dependent upon the effects of nicotine. The return of a normal sense of taste and smell is a pleasure. The improvement in one's skin and general appearance is also a pleasure. The sense of becoming healthier, looking better, smelling nicer, and the pure joy of being able to smell and taste food are all compensation for the occasional urge to smoke.

In people who were heavily addicted, the days of smoking sometimes return in dreams that continue for months. These dreams usually fade with time and eventually cease altogether.

THE FINAL PHASE

The positive results of non-smoking begin to take over after a few weeks or months, depending on the length and intensity of the addiction. Now ex-smokers enter a new phase. Not only do they not crave cigarettes, but they begin to object strongly to cigarette smoke around them. In their place of work, in restaurants, in airplanes, they do not hesitate to make their objection to cigarette smoke known.

The positive effects begin to show. There is an overall sense of greater fitness and health. The shortness of breath disappears, the coughing in the morning is gone, and the aging process that was accelerated by smoking, the "smoker's face," regresses to various extents depending on the age of the ex-smoker and the number of years of smoking. There is a new feeling of health and beauty that had been drowned in a cloud of smoke for many years.

Now food tastes better, and some people do not need to oversalt or overflavor as they used to when their sense of taste was dulled by the smoke and nicotine. The ex-smoker enjoys the fragrance of flowers in blossom in a way that was impossible before. The stale odor of smoke in clothes or old curtains in the house from the smoking days becomes unbearable. It becomes unpleasant if not intolerable to ride in a car where the upholstery smells of smoke. Most ex-smokers cannot go into a hotel room where smokers have been: They are more sensitive to the smell of stale smoke than people who have never smoked. It's interesting that most of these people did not have this sensitivity in their smoking days.

When these positive effects begin, smokers know that their attempts to become ex-smokers have succeeded. They have an inner confidence that their smoking days are gone forever.

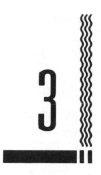

CONCERNS AND QUESTIONS
OF EX-SMOKERS

WHAT ABOUT DEPRESSION AFTER QUITTING?

Some ex-smokers go through a period of anxiety and have some difficulty functioning normally during the first week or two after quitting, but most people don't get depressed. That statement does not alter the fact that nicotine is a stimulant and that the absence of that stimulant may leave some people with a sense of torpor and lethargy, in effect a sense of mild depression. But the lack of a familiar stimulant is significantly different from severe clinical depression requiring professional psychological help or anti-depressant drugs. The lack of this stimulant *can be* a problem for creative people who use the "brain hit" of nicotine to move their brain into high gear. Fortunately this dependency also passes, especially when exercise (an excellent antidote) takes over.

However, given how common depression is in adults, ex–cigarette smokers who later become depressed are susceptible to relapse just as alcoholics are, because depressed people don't care much about anything, including their personal health. That may prompt them to start smoking again. It may help to keep in mind that smoking only makes life more difficult by leaving a person who's already feeling sad and angry to cope with all the hassles of nicotine addiction again. Certainly a feeling of depression in an ex-smoker should be a strong signal to seek professional help and not just "fight it out."

WHAT ABOUT RELAPSE AFTER MANY SMOKE-FREE YEARS?

What leads to relapse after many years without direct exposure to nicotine? It is often the memory of what cigarette smoking did for them when they were sad, tense, or anxious. There is a temptation to fall back on old habits for comfort. Many people feel that since they have conquered their addiction so well, one cigarette won't restart the cycle. This is seldom true: Most of the time that one cigarette means the ex-smoker will soon smoke a pack or two a day. This is true in many other types of addiction as well.

Most people who have stopped smoking and have taken up the habit again will say that they lost their will-power. Some psychologists say there is no such thing as willpower; rather, there are simply certain skills that need to be learned to control behavior. They don't like the word *willpower* because it implies some mystical property that can't be measured. But in practical terms we still need to understand that when people say that they have lost their willpower they mean they've lost a sense of control over their lives. They have been carrying an image of themselves as non-smokers, and if they suffer relapse, they may feel that their life is starting to fall apart. People who lose their self-esteem, confidence, and optimism are more inclined to return to behavior that has comforted them in the past, to go back to an old, familiar habit, even when they know it isn't good for them. They lose their self-respect, and that includes the respect for their bodies.

WHAT ABOUT ALCOHOL?

The combination of alcohol and stress may lead ex-smokers down the path to relapse. Alcohol releases both social and personal inhibitions, which helps undermine the ex-smoker's determination. Though initially a stimulant—alcohol makes people feel reckless and carefree—subsequently it is a depressant, making people feel that it doesn't matter what they do. Neither of those feelings is helpful to ex-smokers, who need to keep their wits about them to resist the temptation to light up "just this once." "Just this once" is the signpost that marks the road back to smoking.

WHAT ABOUT CRAVING SWEETS?

There is another side effect of nicotine addiction: When people stop smoking they develop a passion for sugar. In one study, those who gained weight responded to the increased desire for sugar by eating more sweets without increasing their exercise. Ex-smokers have to be careful about increasing the number of calories they consume from sugar, particularly since many sweets are combined with calorie-laden fats in foods like chocolate, doughnuts, and ice cream.

It's best to try to satisfy the craving for sweets with the natural sugars found in fresh fruits. Fruit also satisfies the desire for oral gratification and answers the need to find something to do with your hands. Fruits that need peeling—oranges, tangerines, tangelos, and bananas, for example—serve all three purposes. They also increase your carbohydrates and fiber, so you can feel doubly virtuous. Besides, it's practically impossible to get fat eating fresh fruit. You may even *lose* weight, because the fruit provides enough bulk to satisfy your hunger, so you may not eat as much as you did before you quit smoking.

The other alternative to eating sweets is increasing physical activity. Swimming, cycling, and working out with weights all burn calories and keep your hands busy and your thoughts off smoking. Once again, you get to feel virtuous: You've quit smoking *and* you're getting more fit.

WHAT ABOUT WEIGHT GAIN?

Is it true that people gain weight after they quit smoking? How much? Is it inevitable? Can it be prevented? What is its cause? The increased craving for sweets is one reason some ex-smokers gain weight. Once the craving for sweets comes under control, the weight gain can be reversed.

Animal experiments have shown that animals with free access to food lose weight when they are given nicotine. The higher the dose of nicotine, the more weight they lose. It may be that nicotine reduces their appetite. Studies with humans, however, suggest that appetite does *not* decrease among smokers, and that smokers don't consume fewer calories.

Nicotine and other constituents of cigarette smoke are poisons. They are often called metabolic poisons because they affect the basic mechanism of different cells of the body. The way these poisons work is not completely understood. It could be that the human body does not assimilate the calories from food normally, either in the process of digestion or in the transformation of calories to fat. This means that the body cannot use those calories for energy or energy storage. The net result is that people lose weight.

Even though nicotine has these effects on cells of the body, it is not true, fortunately, that weight gain is the norm. In one research project where large numbers of ex-smokers were tested, two-thirds either stayed at the same weight or lost weight. Only one-third of the ex-smokers gained weight, and the average gain was only a few pounds, although for some there was a larger weight gain.

Our culture places such a premium on slimness that often even normal weight is perceived as fat. Both men and women worry about gaining weight but, because our society places a greater importance on women's appearance than on men's, women worry more. Some women refuse to stop smoking because the fear that they will gain weight is so intense.

Even if ex-smokers gain a moderate amount of weight, the risk to their health is far less than the risks inherent in smoking. Those who lose or do not gain weight after quitting smoking often change other aspects of their lives as well. They take the next step toward better health and fitness by choosing foods more carefully and eating more fresh fruits, vegetables, and whole grains, and less high-fat meats and cheeses; they work toward greater fitness by getting more exercise. It is important to make some changes in the diet at the time of quitting if the ex-smoker wants to prevent weight gain. These changes promote good health in many other ways, and the benefits can be substantial.

WHAT ABOUT DEVICES TO PREVENT RELAPSE?

The stories that follow show that people have been successful using a variety of items that give their hands something to do when they would normally be playing with a cigarette. To satisfy the need to have something in your mouth in place of a cigarette, chewing gum and, in the early stages after quitting, even lollipops and other candies may be justified. You'll find other suggestions in the stories in Chapter 4.

In extreme cases some of the drugs, such as nicotine gum, that are used to help people to stop smoking may be useful in preventing relapse.

A final suggestion: In the early stages after quitting, avoid situations that once triggered cigarette smoking. For example, for a few weeks stay away from social events that may be strongly associated with smoking, such as cocktail parties, and don't visit friends who are heavy smokers.

THE VOICES OF
EXPERIENCE: EX-SMOKERS
TELL THEIR STORIES

These are the stories of people (like you) who smoked—until one day they found the key that unlocked the door to freedom from smoking. They are people of all ages and all professions, males and females. Different as their stories are, each with its subtext of upbringing, environment, and social attitudes toward smoking, all have the theme of failure followed by success. See which stories most closely parallel your own smoking pattern. Perhaps you will find the key there.

SAMANTHA G.
I Can Quit Anytime I Want

Samantha G., now sixteen, comes from a family with a long his-
tory of addiction to cigarettes. Her father, aunt, grandfather, and
both grandmothers all smoked heavily at some time in their lives;
all have struggled, with varying degrees of success, to quit.
Samantha began smoking two years ago at age fourteen, just
before she entered ninth grade. She thinks she might give up smok-
ing when it's time for her to start her own family.

While the men and women in all the other stories in this book
have successfully quit smoking, Samantha is the exception; as a
teen-ager, she thinks she can quit whenever she wants to. All the
stories that follow prove that this is not the case: quitting is not
easy, and there can be many relapses.

Before I started smoking I was always saying, "You put
that cigarette out! Na-na-na-na-na! You're gonna die!
Blah-blah-blah-blah-blah." I was totally against it. But
here I am, smoking right now. Yeah, I smoke every day.
A pack lasts me about three or four days. It's not like I'm
going to get cancer next year.

I had my first cigarette at the end of eighth grade. A
friend of mine was smoking and we were walking home,
and I said, "Well, here, let me try one." And I did! And I
liked it. "Give me another one!"

That first time was neat. I don't know if it was the

nicotine, but the first time I smoked it, yeah, it gave me a little head rush. It was like, "Wow!" At first I thought it was a cool thing to do and I'm all, "Hey, give me a smoke." It wasn't like I was smoking constantly. I'd have a few cigarettes, and then maybe two or three weeks would go by and I'd see some friends and they'd have smokes so I'd go, "Can I have a cigarette?" "Well, sure!"

It was fun. Other kids were doing it, and since I was a freshman, I thought, "Well, gee, maybe they'll think more of me if I smoke cigarettes." I thought it was the cool thing to do. (Now it's not cool.)

I never bought a pack of cigarettes until the middle of ninth grade. I'd see friends and I'd say, "Can I have a drag? Give me a drag," but I wouldn't buy a pack 'cause there was no way I was going to smoke the whole thing. I don't do that now. I don't buy a pack, smoke it in two minutes, and go out and buy another pack. A pack'll last me a couple of days—unless I'm at a party and I've given them all out.

My parents won't let me smoke at home. They say the house could go up in flames in a minute, and besides, they're parents, you know. Parents don't want their kids to smoke cigarettes. They say it's bad for you.

It gets on my nerves—my parents telling me not to smoke in the house like that's going to keep me from smoking anywhere else. I just go outside. I can smoke there, but I can't smoke in the house. That makes me mad because my grandmother smoked in the house for years. She owns it.

Smoking relaxes me. I can do my homework easier. I

can sit down calmly and do my homework instead of sitting there looking at my homework thinking, "I don't wanna do this." It's not a hundred percent difference. It just makes me go "Aaahhh." It's like a baby with a bottle. You know, when a baby is crying and it starts sucking a bottle and it shuts up. But since I can't smoke when I do my homework, I don't get my homework done!

A bunch of my friends smoke, but there're some who don't like it. Then there are some who say they've quit and then I'm all, "When did you quit?" "Yesterday." And then they'll ask me for a cigarette. That's a worthless cause. I only do it because it's something to do. But it gives me bad breath so I carry Certs or something with me.

My dad quit smoking. He's straight. He won't touch anything now. He doesn't drink or smoke or anything. He goes to A.A. a lot.

If my parents bought me a car, I would quit in a minute. Nothing like a pair of shoes or something; a pair of shoes is gone in a month, but a car would last me. If they give me a car, I'll quit! And if the car breaks down, I'll get it fixed, because once I quit smoking, I probably wouldn't start again. Hopefully. Knock on wood.

I don't smoke instead of eating. There'll be days when I'll have a couple pieces of fruit, and nothing else, and smoke, but it's not like I'm smoking to become anorexic. But that's not every day. There'll be days when I pork out, you know? Sometimes I get mad and I think, "I know, I'll go eat some food." And then the next day I'll go, "Uuuhh," and then just sit and smoke cigarettes.

49

If I'm pissed off, I'll smoke a pack, but I'm usually not pissed off 'cause it's summertime right now. I get pissed off when my parents get on my nerves, or if it's a gloomy day, or if it rains. I don't like the rain.

I usually have a cigarette in the morning around nine or something and then about three o'clock. Every day, I have one in the morning, and then at lunch, and then after school, and then the rest of the day I'll have a cigarette here and there. After school I go out with my friends and we'll all be smoking cigarettes. I go to a store to buy them.

When I'm out of school, I can see myself smoking once in a while. But I want to have a family, which means I'm gonna have to stop, because it's very dangerous if you're pregnant and you smoke. There is no way I am going to smoke when I am having kids. I know I'll quit smoking by then. Until then, who knows?

When my grandmother smoked, it didn't upset me except when we'd be eating dinner, and she would be smoking, and she'd have three cigarettes in the fifteen minutes. That was really sick. I don't smoke when I eat a meal. I'll have one afterwards, because okay, you're full, no more. Here, relax. Have a cigarette. But my grandmother did it before, during, and after, and it was so disgusting. She had cartons everywhere.

Older people do it because they're addicted. And they've probably been smoking for a long time. Or their parents did it, or brothers or sisters, or their husbands or wives.

They keep doing it because it is too hard to quit. My

other grandmother quit smoking at sixty-seven. She shouldn't have done it because she's really heavy and she's got bad arthritis, and when she stopped smoking she gained a lot of weight. And it was like, "Well, why are you doing it now?" Not to say, "Why are you doing it now, you're not gonna live much longer," but, "Why are you doing it now, because it won't make much difference."

I think she would be better right now if she was still smoking, because then she wouldn't have gained as much weight as she did. That's not good because she's got bad arthritis, and she's going to have to have surgery on her knees. And it's kind of sad, too. Also, I love her.

But I don't think I'll be smoking then, because, like I said, if I am going to have a family, I don't want to be smoking. I don't want my kids saying, "Mommy, what are you doing? Mommy, stop smoking!" Or if I had a lot of kids: "Mom, gimme a cigarette!"

I wouldn't want to smoke around my kids. Little kids should not be brought up with smoke because they're so alive with energy. And they might start smoking at an earlier age than me.

I don't think I have cancer yet. I mean, I shouldn't— I've only been smoking about a year and a half.

AMANDA M.
Nicotine Slavery

Amanda M., now thirty-seven, studied modern dance in New York and worked for many years as a dancer and choreographer. Later, she pursued her dance career on the West Coast until an injury forced her to retire. She has embarked on a new career in advertising. She used to worry, after seventeen years as a smoker, that she wouldn't be able to dance if she stopped smoking.

When I was smoking and living in New York, I would go out on a Saturday night, come home at two in the morning, and realize I was out of cigarettes. I'd pick butts out of my ashtray or trash can and smoke them. You know, with coffee stains or bits of food or lipstick on them. It was nicotine slavery!

Nobody is born needing to smoke. Nobody starts out needing to be a drug addict. You do it to yourself. I remember in high school thinking, "God, how disgusting! How could anybody ever even want to smoke? And what would that wanting to smoke feel like? I can't imagine such a weird thing." The first cigarette I ever smoked was in my junior year in high school. I smoked one or two, thought it was stupid, and stopped doing it. All the other kids in my school were doing it, so I thought I should try it. It was horrible. It tasted disgusting, and it made me shiver and shudder.

I didn't smoke again until I was in Czechoslovakia on a trip with a group from my prep school. It was a very loosely arranged two-month tour of Europe. My best friend was on the trip with me. She was five-foot-ten, thin and slinky, and very glamorous. And she smoked! I wanted to emulate her.

I would smoke a couple of cigarettes, come home, and lie in front of the TV feeling nauseous. I don't know why I kept doing it. I guess I thought I was being risqué. And, more importantly, I was doing something my parents absolutely forbade.

Nobody in my family smoked. Never. They were always ranting about it. My grandfather died of emphysema from smoking in 1970. And my father is a pathologist. My parents are against it because they're health-conscious people and they know that smoking can kill you. My father had smoked in the forties and fifties and had quit. It wasn't a struggle for him. He just quit.

Neither my brother nor my sister has ever smoked a single cigarette. I'm the oldest. I smoked as an act of rebellion against my family. I was eighteen and getting seriously into adolescent angst and rebellion. I wanted to assert my independence. Still, it wasn't exactly open rebellion: In seventeen years of smoking I never once lit a cigarette in front of my parents.

All my friends smoked in college. We sat around and smoked cigarettes, middle-class girls sitting around being sullen, hating the establishment and objecting to the war in Vietnam. We smoked and talked and stayed up much too late. And we smoked a lot when we studied and stayed up all night for exams. We all knew smoking was bad for us, but it was somehow like thumbing our noses at the rules, particularly since our parents said it was horrible.

We smoked cigarettes, smoked pot, and took Dexedrine so we could stay awake and talk some more. We spent endless hours philosophizing about life. I associated smoking with thinking deeply and being intellectual.

I had an eating disorder where I would get really uptight or mad, or something wouldn't turn out well, and I'd think, "*I* don't care. I'll just eat. I'll be ugly and stupid and eat up all this stuff." I would eat too much, get furious with myself, and then smoke to kill my appetite, so I wouldn't binge any more.

When I graduated I said, "Ah, now I can quit smoking because life is going to be ever so much simpler now that I'm not in school any more. All my troubles are over." Now that seems kind of a funny statement! I moved to New York, and of course, living there was more a panic than anything else I had ever experienced.

I worked in offices during the day. I'd get bored and I'd smoke out of boredom. In the evening I had dance classes at the studio, and all the dancers smoked waiting for class to start and then they'd smoke after class, cooling down. New York is a smoking culture.

Those were the days when some dance teachers smoked while they were teaching. I don't think they are allowed to now. I think all of the ones who did are dead. I do! They don't do that any more.

Dancers smoke partially to not eat, I think. A lot of dancers have poor eating habits, particularly ballet dancers, and smoking has a lot to do with not wanting to eat. And partially it's something to do to kill time at rehearsals while you're waiting for your turn to dance. That was in New York. And if you live in New York City the air is so polluted, you honestly wonder what difference smoking is going to make. In California, hardly anybody in dance smokes. I can't think of anybody who does. Being a dancer is very stressful. You're always exhausted, you're always running around trying to whip together dance concerts, rehearsing, going to class, and working some miserable daytime job as a secretary or waitress so you can pay the rent and buy groceries. I saw myself as a groovy dancer or *artiste*—a New York *artiste*—not as self-destructive but as committed to creating art.

I worked in a publishing house as an editorial assistant five hours a day. I rehearsed in the afternoon, went to class at six o'clock every night, got home about eight-thirty, and had dinner. I usually went out because I was too tired to cook. I would end up eating hamburgers, stay out smoking and talking, talking and partying. And I'd drink, and smoke.

Every time I smoked I'd think, "This is really stupid. Why are you doing this? This could kill you. Why are you doing this? It's gonna make you wrinkled. It'll make you go through early menopause. It will make you old, and stinky, and ugly. Why are you doing this?" But I wasn't ready to stop, I guess. The little voice that tells you to stop hadn't spoken and said, "No! Enough!"

I never took drugs after college, but I smoked when I was bored or nervous or happy or having fun. Or because I was mad. Smoking blocks out emotions. If I got upset about something, I wanted to have a cigarette. It puts a lid on things and takes away the immediacy of what you're feeling.

The first time I tried to quit, I was living in Minneapolis, not New York. I wasn't dancing. I was living in a nicer place, and I wasn't as nervous as I used to be. That's basically what it was. There were still a number of people around who smoked, but there were also women I knew who had smoked about as long as I had who were quitting or who had quit recently. That's what motivated me to think about quitting, but my attempts to quit were half-hearted. I would always cheat.

I said, "This is for the birds," and I signed up for a quit-smoking class, and I went, and I *still* cheated. I never really stopped smoking. I would smoke, maybe, two cigarettes a day. I had all these signs—"Thank you for not smoking"—and brochures about smoking and all sorts of charts, stuff that's part of a packet of non-smoking material they give you when you sign up for the class. I did cut down for a couple of months. Way down. But then I started smoking more, and as soon as I allowed myself to do it once, I did it again. And again. I became lax, and gradually, over a week or two, I was smoking.

I went back to smoking my habitual amount, fifteen to twenty cigarettes a day. I think everybody has a different level of how much they will smoke, given free rein. My limit was about a pack a day. Some people smoke two packs a day, some people smoke three packs a day. It is incomprehensible to me that anybody could stand to smoke that much.

The man I was living with also smoked, but he didn't have any compulsion to smoke, as I did. He smoked mostly to be social. He could go out to a party, smoke a pack, and not smoke again for three days. We had our own apartment, and we both smoked. Then he quit. We went to see his parents and his father is a very heavy smoker. He quit because it made him sick to see his father smoking. Then he would tell me not to smoke in the car when he was in it. I would do what he asked because I knew it was annoying, but I still smoked at home.

Then we moved to California into a group house where they had a rule: no smoking in the house. We did it on purpose. But since I couldn't smoke in the house, I went out in the backyard to smoke instead.

At the same time, I quit drinking coffee, which made it much easier for me not to smoke in the morning. I used to stagger to the coffee pot, smoke while I waited for the coffee to drip, and have a cigarette or two with my coffee.

I smoked at work still. I was a secretary in San Francisco, at two different corporations. And I started dancing again. There were only one or two other people who smoked in the class. It wasn't the same kind of studio atmosphere as in New York, where everybody hangs out in the studio and smokes. In California you go to class, take the class, and go home. I didn't have all my smoking friends here. It wasn't the same at all.

A year before I quit smoking, that guy Latka on "Taxi"

died of lung cancer, but it wasn't from smoking. He was only one year older than I was, and that really gave me the creeps. I was thirty-four—and he died of lung cancer! I thought, "Oh, God, this is horrible. He is only a little bit older than me and he has died of this weird cancer." From that day I made a rule that I could smoke no more than six cigarettes a day.

Then they passed the law in San Francisco that said you couldn't smoke in an office building unless you had a private office with a door. That cut my smoking down even more.

It was hard at first, because it's such a habit. It's like not exercising when you're used to exercise. You feel like, "Eeyuchh!" You want to scream or something. I'd get nervous and irritable, and I'd want to stuff my face. I'd drink diet pop or eat Cheetos. I got used to it, though.

I read a lot of quit-smoking books, and one really got to me. It talked about all of the physiological changes that one cigarette causes in your body. It was amazing. Worse, it said that you can smoke about 100,000 cigarettes and not necessarily cause permanent physical damage, but after that, with each one you smoke, you're playing Russian roulette, because that one could give you cancer or emphysema or heart disease. *That one.* Reading that did it, because I was sure I had probably smoked that many. I was sick of smoking. It was a pain to deal with it any more.

I still had a studio in New York, where I had my things in storage. I decided I wasn't going to live there, so I went back to arrange for everything to be shipped to

California. I was still smoking my six cigarettes or less a day that I started when that guy on "Taxi" died.

At JFK Airport, waiting for my flight back to California, I had one cigarette left in the pack. I smoked it, crumpled up the pack, and said, "That's that!" And that *was* that. I didn't decide ahead of time. The day came when it was time to stop, and I stopped. Perhaps I associated it with closing the chapter on my life in New York, my years of adolescent rebellion, my image of myself as the driven *artiste.* I was leaving all of that stuff behind.

I used the things I learned in the quit-smoking class in Minneapolis—the signs and things they gave me. I put one up on my desk at home, and I put one up at work. They were sort of boosterish messages to myself. They say, "Thank you for not smoking," and I would say to myself, "Thank you for not smoking." Every time I looked at them, I would thank myself.

I didn't get nauseous and throw up, or get constipated, but I was nervous and wanted to eat. Every night I ate a giant bowl of popcorn with no butter, a huge bowl of popcorn. I would sit there and stuff my face with it around nine or ten at night. I did it every night for six months. Then I did it about three nights a week. And then about six months ago, I couldn't stand the sight of popcorn any more.

Now that I've stopped smoking, I feel better. When I drank coffee and smoked I was very sluggish when I got up. Now I just wake up and I'm awake. I can even have a normal conversation within three minutes of getting up.

It's like being a kid. I don't drink any stimulants like coffee or caffeine tea when I get up. I just drink water and leave the house and I'm fine.

I haven't noticed food tasting better or smelling things more, but my clothes smell better, and I smell better. And I have much better color. I used to get really pale, and I think it was from smoking. When I first was in New York, my cheeks would get rosy when I danced, and after seven years of smoking, they didn't. My wind is obviously much better. I used to get winded going up the stairs for a subway, even though I danced hours every week.

I had always been very interested in health and nutrition. I always ate basically healthy food—broiled chicken, steamed broccoli, and baked potatoes. There were things that I ate then that I wouldn't eat now. Candy and cake and coffee, for example.

I didn't drink at all when I first quit because I couldn't separate the two in my mind; they really went together. Now I drink wine, but I don't need to smoke when I do it. I don't even think about it any more. I just don't smoke.

I thought that choreographing without smoking would be a problem, but it wasn't. When I moved out here no smoking was allowed in dance studios, so even though I was still smoking, I couldn't smoke when I was in the studio. I adapted to the situation. I used to worry that I wouldn't be able to dance and choreograph any more, the way writers quit smoking sometimes and think they can't write without a cigarette hanging out of their mouth, but it's not a problem.

I used to think about having a cigarette every day, but

every time I wanted to smoke I'd say to myself, "Just wait it out, it'll pass." And I'd get over it. I'd go for a walk, exercise, or do long stretches and wait until the moment passed. That's how I did it: As the urge came to smoke, I would wait until it passed. They became farther and farther apart, and I thought about smoking less and less. Now, most of the time, I never think about smoking, unless someone is smoking near me, and then I get disgusted. I hate it and I don't let anybody ever smoke in the house where I live. I hate the way it smells, and it makes me feel like I'm choking: It's as simple as that!

I always was a weird smoker. I couldn't be in smoky bars for very long because the smoke hurt my eyes. It was very difficult—my eyes would get red and burn. And if I had gone for twenty-four hours without smoking, the first time I would smoke a cigarette would give me those shudders. I mean it physically affected me in a disgusting way.

When I was smoking six or less a day, every time I smoked I could feel the hit. I could feel my heart rate increase, and I could feel myself getting wired. The physiological things were as plain as day. It's the same thing that coffee does to me.

Smoking always seemed like it wasn't me. As I became an adult, I started associating smoking with people who were uneducated, who didn't know any better, who didn't take responsibility for their health. I felt weird about smoking toward the end. I thought, "This is a creepy thing to be doing." I was embarrassed that I did it. I felt humiliated at myself. I wasn't feeling very good about myself in general, and so these feelings about smoking reinforced my lousy self-image as an inadequate twit. Somebody who wasn't quite with it. Somebody who wasn't successful.

I feel tremendously clean from not smoking. Now I see myself as an energetic person who is bright and fun to be around, somebody who's disciplined and had the strength to quit smoking.

Every once in a while I'll just get this flash: "Gee! I'd like a cigarette." I get them at all different times. I'll be driving down the street and all of a sudden have this feeling of wanting to smoke, or be talking to somebody and want to smoke. I just put it out of my mind.

After I quit, I dreamed about coughing up blood. I was coughing and there was blood on my pillow. I dreamt it twice. I never dreamed about it while I was smoking, but after I quit I did. It gives me the creeps.

My ex-boyfriend started smoking again. He asked me, "Don't you ever sneak a puff or anything?" No. I never do. I never will, because I can't. I was addicted to nicotine. And he is, too.

Sometimes I feel weak when something horrible has happened. I had another boyfriend who turned out to be a terrible jerk. I was really upset, and I talked to a friend of mine and I said, "I feel like having a cigarette." She said, "Don't do it; he's not worth it. Nothing is worth it. Don't do it." Every time I'm really upset about something and I find myself thinking, "I want to smoke," I think instead, "It's not worth it. This piece-of-shit person is not *worth* smoking over. This ridiculous work situ-

ation isn't *worth* smoking over. It's no big deal, ₁
going to die—except me, if I start smoking again.

JAMES V.
Pictures of Smokers' Lungs

James V., in his late fifties, has been a truck driver for thirty years, delivering tons of gravel to construction sites. The roads are sometimes steep, the traffic is often heavy, and the trucks are always loaded to their legal limit of 80,000 pounds. As James says, "You don't want to hit anybody because these big trucks kill people real easy." Even the dumping must be done with care and skill to keep the truck from overturning.

I started smoking when I was eighteen years old—just about the time I went into the Navy in 1950. I enlisted to go to Korea and started smoking when I was in training in San Diego.

In the service they used to have a saying, "The smoking lamp is lit," and whenever they told you that, you could stop and smoke. Or if there was a coffee shop nearby, you could have coffee and smoke. All of that kind of goes together. Even if you didn't smoke when you went in, you'd probably start in the service. My brother, who didn't smoke until he was almost twenty-five, started smoking in the service.

In the beginning, smoking would make me dizzy. If I went without smoking for too long, maybe a few hours, and then took a drag on a cigarette, I'd get dizzy. Pretty soon the dizziness was over and I'd feel all numb—almost like taking a drink.

In my smoking days, I remember there were spots along the road, certain places where the truck goes slow, and I'd take out a cigarette and light it and smoke it while I went up the hill. Then thirty or forty minutes later I'd have to have another one. I'd get the craving, and there'd be another spot on the highway for the next smoke. I'd been doing that since I started driving in 1958.

When I first started, I smoked Lucky Strikes with no filter, and then after my grandfather died—he was a heavy smoker—I started smoking filter cigarettes. I started with filters as soon as they came out. Later I switched to True—less nicotine, less tar, and all of that baloney. They're supposed to do you less harm. Well, I talked my wife into smoking them too, but now she smokes more than she did before, because she gets less out of them. I was the same way—you just smoke more cigarettes.

I was raised as a Seventh Day Adventist. I went to religious schools up to high school, and I didn't believe in smoking or drinking or theaters or even hardly holding hands with girls, so I was raised up real strict. But when I thought I was old enough, and I was on my own, I figured I could do what I wanted. Nobody could tell me what to do. I was rebelling against my folks and religion. I quit going to the church, and I started smoking and drinking and chasing girls.

My folks never smoked, either one of them, because of

their religion, and because they didn't think they should. They said smoking was bad even back then, but they didn't tell us why. They just said it was bad. And I figured, well, it's because of their religion—that's why.

I was about eighteen when I started and I was thirty-three when I realized that my relatives were dying because of their smoking habit. None of them were Seventh Day Adventists like my mother and father. My grandfather died and my uncle and another uncle, and they all smoked and smoked and smoked since they were little children. They came from the Midwest, where tobacco was plentiful. They all died young: My grandfather died when he was sixty-four; one uncle died of a stroke when he was around sixty; and another one died from lung cancer around sixty-two. I realized then that, "Hey, something's wrong, something is causing that." So I decided to quit when I was in my early thirties.

I was driving trucks then, too. As I've said, that's quite stressful. I realized how much better I felt the first time I quit. It takes a little while to start feeling better. For a while you still have that great desire, but you have to overpower it mentally, you have to think it away.

Nobody told me I should quit: I decided I had better quit or I would end up like my grandfather and my uncles, and so I did quit—I just made up my mind one day. I had tried to quit quite a few times before that, but after a few days I would sneak a cigarette and think, "It won't hurt me." I would have a drag, start to smoke the cigarette, and it would make me dizzy, so I would put it out, but after a while it breaks your will down. I would say,

"Well, I've already had one, so I might as well try another one," and pretty soon I'd try another one ten hours later, and the next day I'd try another one. Within a day or two I'd buy another pack and put it back in my pocket and I was hooked again. You can't fool yourself, that nicotine makes you want more.

Finally I said, "Well, this is no good." You can't cheat; with smoking, there is no cheating. So I said, "This is it. This is the last one, and no more." After I quit, I would wake up in the morning, and no cigarette, and I would fight all day long with myself mentally.

I did not smoke for nine years. Then my first wife and I split up after nineteen years of marriage. She pulled away, she left me. I was about forty-one. After the divorce, the stress was kind of heavy. I started drinking more, and I was so emotionally upset, I didn't care whether I lived or died. I was really in love with her. After nine years I started smoking again and kept smoking clear up until last year.

The reason I quit this time is that my lungs started hurting me. I was hurting, and I could tell I wasn't normal. I would take a deep breath and I would get dizzy. I went to a lung cancer specialist and had my lungs X-rayed and checked for cancer, and I went to a throat specialist and had my throat checked out for cancer. It all came out negative, but I decided, "Well, that's it. I am not taking no more chances, because I'm no kid no more, and it can catch up with me." So I quit, and I had to fight the desire to smoke again—just like it was the first time I quit.

It took about six months, but the first few days were the worst. And then gradually, the craving gets less and less. Your system gets used to not having the nicotine. Now I hardly crave it at all.

The wife I am married to now smokes a whole bunch. She smokes about two or three packs a day. She is quite a bit younger than I am, but if she is going to smoke, she is going to smoke. I can't stop her. Everybody has to quit themselves, if they want to. I don't nag her. I let her do what she wants to do. I just told her, "I hate to see you kill yourself like that, but it will happen if you keep going. I have seen too much of it." I stick right with her, whether she smokes or not.

Now I snack quite a bit, but I try to snack on health foods, like cereals. Once in a while I get a package of peanuts or sunflower seeds—it gives me something to do with my hands. When I first quit, I started doing that—it gets your mind off cigarettes, because you're sitting there picking shells off sunflower seeds or peanuts.

I used to dream a lot when I first quit. I'd dream I was smoking, and it would scare me when I woke up because I thought I had been smoking, which I hadn't been. You'd wake up and say, "What's happened here?" Then you realize you didn't smoke and you're real glad, real happy.

Another thing that helped me to quit this last time were these colored pictures I saw somewhere of a good, non-smoking lung and of a smoker's lung. The smoker's lung looked like a roast beef compared with the non-smoker's lung. You could hardly tell what it was from the pictures. On the good lung you could see everything very plain, but the smoker's lung looked like it was cooked.

It has been a year this spring since I quit. One of my uncles passed away at that time. Before he passed away, he would come and stay at my house for a few days. When he came back last time he was complaining of hurting and hurting and hurting. He had been a smoker since he was six years old, and he was sixty-five when he died. He only lived with me a few months before he died. He wouldn't talk very much, he would just say, "I'm hurting." He couldn't eat hardly any food. I said, "Well, you got to eat," and I took him to my doctor, who said, "He's got lung cancer," so they gave him cobalt treatments and the cobalt treatments hurt him bad. The day before he died, he wanted a cigarette, so I went and got him some cigarettes. I had quit by then. He helped me make up my mind that I had better stay off cigarettes because I had seen too much of what they can do with him and his brothers and his dad.

My mother passed away last year just after I quit smoking and she was eighty-two. My dad is eighty-four now, and he is still going strong. He's got good lungs and a good mind and he is still all together. He was a non-smoker. My mother's brothers are the ones who died young, and her father died young, and they were all smokers. My wife's mother has one sister who is a non-smoker and she is still going good, but she has another sister who is about to die, and she is a smoker. To me, that is proof in my mind as to what smoking will do to you. It is all black and white in my own family—the ones that don't smoke live a long life and the ones that do smoke die young. That tells me a lot.

Something else has helped me to quit. I listen to the radio every day going down the highway from one until two in the afternoon. I listen to this doctor, Dr. Dean Edell, as he talks about the hazards of smoking, and addiction to smoking, and how heavy a drug it is, and how they have come out recently that smoking is just as hard to quit as heroin. They say if you can quit smoking, and if you're a druggie or an alcoholic, you can quit any of them, because smoking is the toughest one to quit. He has helped me; I have listened to him for years. He helped encourage me a little bit, and then my uncle dying, that really encouraged me.

DAVID GOERLITZ
The Winston Man

For six years, David Goerlitz was the Winston Man, the model who represented Winston cigarettes in newspaper and magazine advertising. He was a three-pack-a-day smoker who smoked Winstons and was proud of it. When he gave up smoking, he stopped modeling for Winston—and walked away from $75,000 a year in doing so. Figuring that he persuaded many young people to start smoking in his years as the Winston Man, he is now committed to persuading people to stop. He is thirty-nine years old.

Doesn't it seem odd to you that 95 percent of the people who die of lung cancer are smokers? Or that 78 percent of the people who die of heart disease are smokers? It's a horrible feeling to be aware of what cigarettes do to people's health, knowing that I was the main reason that Winston became the number-two-selling cigarette over a four-year period. I have a very guilty conscience about that.

I loved smoking, loved it. I didn't just light cigarettes; I *smoked* them. I wasn't even out of bed when I had my first cigarette. The first thing I did in the morning was smoke a cigarette; the last thing I did at night was smoke a cigarette. I started when I was fifteen, and I smoked for twenty-four years. I was up to three and a half packs a day when I quit.

There wasn't a day that went by that I didn't smoke. It didn't matter if I had a cold, I smoked. When I was in the hospital with my whole left side paralyzed, I smoked. I was working as Harrison Ford's double in *Witness*, doing stunts, and the last week of the shoot, my left side suddenly became paralyzed. They gave me VIP treatment in the hospital, complete with a private room, and in my room I could do anything I wanted, including smoke. The first thing I did in the morning was smoke a cigarette, and the last thing I did in the evening was smoke a cigarette.

The evidence of addiction became more and more undeniable as I got older. I would not go to sleep if I was down to fewer than ten or twelve cigarettes. I would go out and buy a pack of cigarettes so I'd have them in case I woke up in the night and needed them. That *never* happened, but the fear that it *might* only grew stronger as the years went by. I would literally get out of bed on a cold night, get dressed, shovel the snow off my car, and go out to find a store that was open twenty-four hours a day to buy a pack of cigarettes, to be sure those cigarettes were there, just in case.

I used to hide cigarettes under the seats of my car. If I had a pack of cigarettes in my pocket that only had four or five cigarettes left, I'd take that pack and put it under the seat of the car and put a fresh pack in my pocket. I'd store them up just the way a little chipmunk or pack rat would do. I didn't care if they got stale; it didn't matter.

I would go through ashtrays to find a butt that had maybe as much as an inch of tobacco left in it, and I would save those, too. I hoarded them against an emergency, against the day I might need them. I wish I were as good with my money as I was with my cigarettes. I always knew where my cigarettes went, and I always knew where to find some when I needed them.

For twenty-four years I smoked. For four years the neurosurgeon told me I'd better lay off the cigarettes because of the paralysis I had. That didn't stop me. My son, who's now ten, begged me every year on his birthday to stop smoking as his birthday present. That didn't stop me. My mother sent me pictures of tar-coated lungs in the mail. That didn't stop me. My gums had been bleeding for four years, and everyone in my family complained about the way I smelled from smoking. That didn't stop me either.

What stopped me was seeing kids twelve and thirteen buying cigarettes and lighting up, and the fear that I might have influenced them to smoke. What stopped me was the realization that the tobacco industry commits murder, and I have been an accessory for six years. The tobacco industry is pushing a substance as addictive as cocaine or heroin that kills 400,000 people every year from diseases *directly* related to smoking.

Smoking-related diseases are the biggest public health issue in the United States today. Not AIDS. Not drugs. Not even highway deaths. More people die every year from smoking-related diseases than from any other single cause in this country's history, with the exception of World War II. The Surgeon General has declared that secondhand smoke causes lung cancer, and women who don't smoke but whose husbands do have a 40 percent greater chance of getting lung cancer than women who are married to men who don't smoke.

There are 50 million smokers in the United States. That's 26 percent of the population. Every year it's decreased by 4–5 percent. The 4–5 percent who quit are over forty years of age. Look at the figures. Fifty million smokers spending $2 per day is $100 million per day, $700 million per week. The tobacco industry generates $15 *billion* per year. To maintain those kinds of revenues the tobacco industry needs to recruit 5,000 new smokers every single day to offset those who quit—and those who die. The tobacco industry would rather addict the young. They'll be customers longer. That's why cigarette advertising is aimed at teen-agers.

I also feel guilty about having been an inconsiderate smoker. I honestly felt that non-smokers who asked me not to smoke were infringing on my civil rights. "I can smoke if I want to; it's not illegal!" was my resentful reaction. I didn't care about the non-smoker, second-hand smoke, the offensive smell, or any of that stuff.

Now it seems to me that the tobacco companies use the "right to smoke" issue as a diversionary tactic. If smokers and non-smokers fight with each other, maybe they'll never notice that smokers are paying for the dubious privilege of allowing the tobacco companies to reap huge profits from systematically poisoning their customers. Any other industry that did that would be shut down instantly and ordered to pay heavy damages to those who were sick and to the families of those who died.

I have three children in the public schools. They are exposed every day to secondhand smoke from teachers who smoke. Not one of my children smokes, but all of them are exposed to nicotine addiction from their teachers' smoking. The dangers are all clearly detailed in the Surgeon General's 1986 report *Health Effects of Secondary Smoke.* Not to mention the simple hypocrisy of the teachers coming back from their cigarette break and telling the kids to "just say no." I think the 74 percent of us who don't smoke should protect our children's health by making it illegal to smoke anywhere on school property.

I've had great things happen since I stopped smoking. For one thing, I have much more self-esteem and confidence, and that makes my work better. I lost eleven pounds. And I used to worry that sex wouldn't be the same without a cigarette after. I was right; it's not the same. It's better!

TONY B.
I Quit Cold, and That Was It

Tony B., sixty-six, has recently retired as vice-president of CBS Entertainment Productions at CBS Television. One of the pioneers of early television programs, he started out stage-managing, and eventually directing, such live-performance classics as "Playhouse 90," "Studio One," and "Climax." Many of his shows are now considered among the finest ever produced on television.

My mother had a heart attack on Monday. On Tuesday my older brother had a heart attack. On Wednesday my mother died. I was in Los Angeles working in television, and nobody in the family wanted to upset me, so nobody told me what was going on until they called me to come home for my mother's funeral. After going to the funeral, I went to visit my brother, who was so depressed over his condition that nobody had told *him* our mother had died for fear the shock would kill him, too.

I was scared to death. I knew that smoking was bad for me. I'd been thinking about quitting for a long time, but I hadn't done it. When I got back to Los Angeles, I started having chest pains. I kept telling myself it was psychosomatic, that I was making it up because I was upset about my mother and brother. The pains persisted for a couple of weeks, and finally I went to the doctor. He did an examination, and when he was done he said, "Well, of course you're having chest pain. You've had bronchitis for weeks." I almost died of relief.

I reached into my pocket, pulled out my pack of Marlboros, threw them across the desk, and said, "You can have these. I don't need them any more." He laughed, opened his top desk drawer, put them in it, and said, "They'll be here if you decide you want them." I've never touched another cigarette, and that was more than thirty years ago. I had been smoking three packs of cigarettes a day for more than twenty years.

I was uncomfortable for the first three days, and after that the urge just disappeared. I was psychologically prepared for it. That's the key. A person has to be ready to quit smoking, and they have to really want to give it up or need to give it up. I kept thinking to myself, "This is ridiculous. Why should I keep smoking? It's bad for me, it's scaring the hell out of me, and there's no point." I quit cold, and that was it.

I've never had another drag on anything. I don't want to put anything with smoke in my mouth because I *know* that I was addicted. Even now I'm not sure that if I took even one drag that I wouldn't want more. I have no yearning for it, no craving at all, but I just don't want to take the chance.

I dislike it when other people smoke around me, not because it makes me want a cigarette—it doesn't—but because it smells bad. It gets in my hair and on my clothes, and I don't like it.

The real horror, to me, is that the tobacco industry is well aware of how lethal their product is, yet it keeps saying that it's not lethal, that it's okay to smoke, they're putting in filters and there's nothing to worry about. Driven by greed, they continue to foist poison, *real poison*, on the public *knowingly*. That's the horror to me.

Hollywood has a reputation for being stressful and tension-ridden, especially the movie and television industries. You might assume a lot of people in the industry would smoke, but that's not the case. Very few of the people I worked with at CBS or in the studios smoked. They had either quit or never started. For myself, I knew that smoking doesn't relieve tension. That kind of stuff is all in people's heads. I had to learn how to deal with stress in productive ways, not by killing myself.

I jog regularly, and I play a lot of golf. I'm convinced that if I had not quit when I did I wouldn't be able to do the things that I'm doing today. Every time I hear more evidence about how harmful smoking is to the lungs, the heart, the whole cardiovascular system, I thank God that I quit when I did. I'm sure I couldn't enjoy my life as much as I am now if I hadn't quit.

My wife quit smoking a year after I did, and she just came back from a week of whitewater rafting, and a few days later she went backpacking in the Sierras for another week. You can't do that if you can't breathe, or you're worried about your heart.

My brother was only forty-eight when he had his heart attack, and the first thing the doctors told him was to quit smoking. He couldn't do it. Smoking is an addiction. He lived another fourteen years, babying himself so he wouldn't strain his heart and sneaking off to smoke in the bathroom. What a waste, what a *waste.*

MARION R.
I Was a Closet Smoker

Marion R. was born in Austria during World War II. She spent her childhood in convents and private schools. When she was nineteen, she came to the United States and received her higher education here. She was one of the first female computer systems analysts on the East Coast and worked in the computer industry for eight years. Now married, she has two teen-age children and is writing a novel based on her own life. She realizes now how difficult she made her task by constructing private games about her smoking.

I had gone through two years of trying very, very hard to stop smoking, allowing myself only an occasional cigarette here and there. I didn't smoke in the house, I didn't smoke in front of my husband, I didn't smoke around other people. Life became very difficult with all the restrictions I invented for where and when I could smoke. For two years I played these little games with myself, hoping they would help me cut down on my smoking.

What all this really did was to alienate me from other people. I used to disappear so I could have a cigarette while nobody could see me, but they didn't know where

I'd gone or why. It was like being a closet alcoholic—I was a closet smoker. I was embarrassed because I always made this big deal, "I am going to give up smoking," and then didn't. I didn't want anybody to know that I didn't manage it again.

In the end, I didn't sleep well any more—I woke up every night at two o'clock in the morning berating myself, saying, "You worthless human being, why can't you manage to get a better hold of yourself? You can't let cigarettes control your life."

Every night I would say, "Next morning when I get up I won't have a cigarette," and then someplace along the line, I would have one again. I prepared myself seriously for two years to do it, and I half-heartedly quit a couple of times here and there, but that was different from this last time. I went through the whole thing of getting nicotine gum and various and sundry other things as part of my preparations. A couple of times when I had tried to stop previously I had experienced withdrawal symptoms of chills and shaking and being miserable. I imagine that's how it is for alcoholics who stop drinking. This time I got myself ready in case this happened; I had the nicotine gum and everything. One day I chewed a piece of that gum and it was so vile tasting that I said to myself, "Come on . . . you can do without that, can't you?" I chewed the gum for a little while, but that was it. I didn't need the nicotine.

Psychologically, my failures to quit caused me hell. Finally, it was close to my husband's birthday, and I was thinking, "What can I do that is really special?" Although he knew I was smoking, we never talked about it. I decided, "Well, this is it, for myself, for him, for the whole family, for the peace of everybody, I am going to give it up this time and this is going to be it." And I did. It was very simple; it was the easiest quitting episode I have ever had.

I remember so well how it happened. . . . It was the strangest thing; I woke up and I thought, "This is it." Never once in the back of my mind did I even consider sneaking a puff here or there. Overnight, I had the feeling that I was rid of it. The monkey was off my back, and I was not going to smoke ever again. Now I have absolutely no desire to smoke—no desire.

I was not really worried about my health. It wasn't the fear of lung cancer so much, or heart disease. My main reason for wanting to stop smoking was to be in control of myself; the other reasons were all window dressing.

I had smoked for many years before I quit. I began to smoke at thirteen. I thought smoking was very glamorous. Practically every one of my friends smoked—we shouldn't have, but we were really not told not to. I liked smoking right away. I kept on trying to give it up because I couldn't afford cigarettes. There wasn't a lot of money in Austria after the war, and certainly very little for a girl who ran away from home at fourteen. For financial reasons I had to give it up a few times as a teen-ager.

I gave up smoking voluntarily when I became pregnant with each of my children, although it had not been proven at the time that smoking was dangerous to fetuses. By then I was living in the United States. When I had my first child in 1969—I was thirty at that time—I gave up smoking before I became pregnant and didn't smoke for about two and a half years. I guess I thought it was better for pregnant mothers not to smoke. When my son was about eighteen months old, I started smoking again. I had a house guest for two and a half months. She smoked, and having the smoke around me all the time reminded me that I missed it.

The second time around, I gave up smoking before I became pregnant with my second child, in 1972. I kept it up until she got sick when she was a year old. She had to be hospitalized with a terrible flu. I was at the hospital at two in the morning, found a cigarette, and started smoking again. I was terrified of losing my daughter. I was under a lot of stress.

Ever since then I've tried to give it up. I'd quit for two months, or three months or six months, and then I'd fall on my face.

I have always been very athletic, and I found it a bit obscene to be a tennis player hanging around with a cigarette in her hand. I also ride a great deal, and it's very dangerous to have cigarettes around stable areas. I really didn't want to smoke. It frustrated me to keep losing the battle. I hated not wanting to do something but feeling compelled to smoke, hated being addicted to something that I knew was bad for me.

I've tried to quit ten or twelve times in the last twenty years. And very, very rarely did I give up smoking for only a couple of days—I have always given it up for at least two months, most of the time for six to nine months. Every time I went back to smoking, it was as though I had never stopped smoking. I didn't get dizzy, lightheaded, or anything like that, the way it was when I tried smoking the very first time.

About four years ago I had stopped smoking again. For about seven months I did not smoke. I had taken the children skiing and was driving our station wagon at night when I was hit head-on by a drunk driver in a pickup truck. The car spun around, and my head went through the windshield. (The kids weren't hurt, thank heaven.) I had to go to the hospital to have my head sewn up, and as I was recovering the next morning, I thought, "Why am I worrying about the cancer that might kill me if I smoke? Here is this drunken idiot out there who almost killed me, and I'm putting myself through all this agony to stop smoking?" So I started smoking again.

You may wonder why I am so sure this time that I'll never smoke again. Two things are different now. One is that when I stopped before, I used to smoke in my dreams, and I used to wake up hyperventilating from smoking in those dreams. Even when I quit for two and a half years, I used to smoke in my dreams. I have not dreamed that I was smoking since I gave it up this last time, except once. I woke up one night, and I was so disappointed because I dreamed I'd had one puff of a cigarette. It never happened again because I couldn't stand the sense of disappointment.

Something else is different this time. That's how I know I have finally quit at last. For years I went around saying, "Someday I am going to write a book, a novel, but really the story of my life." About two years ago that "someday" arrived. I started off with an outline, did a lot of soul searching, went through a lot of emotional pain, agony, pleasure, exhilaration, a lifetime-size bundle of emotions. I was forced to look at myself in certain ways and didn't feel very comfortable doing it, but I did it anyway. I was able to forgive myself for some of the things I felt I needed to forgive myself for, pat myself on the shoulder for some of the things that I deserved to be patted for. I made peace with some of the figures in my past, made peace with myself partially, and knew that there was no way I could make peace with myself if I let things I didn't like control me—stupid habits like smoking and drinking and such, like little clowns that had a stranglehold on my life.

When I began to write the book two years ago, I began taking the first serious steps toward quitting smoking. I hadn't seen this correlation before, but now that I think about it, it's true. Now that the book is almost finished, I have stopped smoking. The book is the story of my life. I have rediscovered myself by writing the book. That's why I know I'll never smoke again.

DON C.
I Thought It Was Indigestion

Don C. was vice-president of human resources in a major corporation with more than 600 employees when he had a serious heart attack. He and his wife, Mary Jane, have been married thirty-one years. When Don came home from the hospital, Mary Jane was still smoking.

I remember the last day I smoked all too well. It was Labor Day, 1983. I was at home. It was a warm day, the temperature was in the eighties, and I felt extremely hot and tired. In the morning I had had some chest pains that I thought were indigestion. There was a cord of firewood in the driveway to be stacked, there was some shrubbery to clear away, and I wasn't looking forward to all this physical work because I just didn't feel good.

I did it anyway, but by late afternoon, when I'd nearly finished it, I realized something was seriously wrong. I began to perspire heavily, and the pain became more intense and spread across my shoulders. I knew I needed to cool off fast, so I put the garden hose over my head and yelled to my wife to get me to the doctor immediately. She took me to an emergency medical clinic. It only took about five minutes to get there, but something was telling me that every minute counted.

I wasn't fully aware of everything that was going on. They took an electrocardiogram, listened to my heart, asked me a few questions, and diagnosed it as a heart attack. They gave me some nitroglycerin and called a cardiologist. They transported me to a large hospital and put me in the coronary intensive care unit. They thought my condition had stabilized when I went into ventricular fibrillation [extremely irregular heartbeat]. It's a good thing the cardiologist was there. I feel to this day that he saved my life. They put tubes up my arm directly into my heart and they had got out those special electric paddles used to get your heart going again after it stops . . . which frightened me. When I heard them ask if there was a priest on duty, I think that frightened me more than anything else.

I remember hearing the beeping sound from the electronic equipment that I was hooked up to. It was beeping rather rapidly . . . but I was not aware of any pain or any serious discomfort, and I had the feeling that this couldn't really be happening to me.

At any rate, there was full blockage in one of the arteries in the upper left part of the heart. I was in the hospital ten days. I finally realized the full scope of the damage that had been done. I went home for six weeks and then returned to the hospital for an angiogram, a way to photograph the arteries of the heart. It showed partial blockage in two other arteries. A week later I underwent triple-bypass surgery on my heart.

All this put sufficient fear in me that I realized I had to change my life-style. Various cardiologists, before and after the surgery, told me that the operation would not do me any good in the long run if I went back to smoking and if I wasn't more careful about what I ate. In the three years before my heart attack I had been eating less meat and cutting down on fried food, but I hadn't gone far enough. I needed to get into a regular exercise program.

Before all this happened I had been trying to cut down on my smoking, was doing a little exercise, and experiencing some angina—chest pain—but I always thought it was indigestion. When I had asked a doctor about it, he told me it was probably indigestion. I had just taken a physical exam six weeks before my heart attack, and so I knew what I needed to do: exercise more, watch my weight, watch what I was eating. But as one of the cardiologists told me later, the blockage in those arteries occurred over a period of years—not in the last six months. And he told me that I had a good chance to live to a ripe old age if I would pay more attention to these things. If I went back to smoking and my old eating habits, he couldn't guarantee anything. I felt as if I had been hit by lightning, and I don't need to be hit by lightning twice.

I have not touched a cigarette or a pipe or anything resembling tobacco since my heart attack. My last cigarette was on that Labor Day, 1983.

Once I experienced the nearness to death during my heart attack, there was absolutely no question in my mind that I would never have a cigarette again. When my children and my wife came to see me in the hospital, I knew that I could not and would not have a cigarette or pipe ever again.

When I got home from the hospital my wife was still a smoker, and the cigarette smoke still smelled good to me. I used to tell smokers around me, "It's all right to smoke; in fact, it kind of smells good." I have since come to very intensely dislike people smoking around me. I don't like people to smoke in my home, in my car, and I certainly don't let people smoke in my office. I dislike, very much, being around smokers.

I had many thoughts when I realized what had happened to me, regarding my life and my priorities in life. I felt inadequate, incompetent, as they say in management. I thought, "Why did this happen to me? I know people who are obese, who smoke much more than I do, who get absolutely no exercise. Why did this happen to me?" I was only five to ten pounds overweight, I was a smoker, but not a heavy smoker, and I just couldn't understand it. I had great concern for my longevity and a high interest in what I needed to do to live to a ripe old age. It made me stop and think about my children, the importance to me of work, the importance of my friends, the quality of my life. These are the things I thought about while I was in the hospital, having little else to do other than stare up at the ceiling.

I had smoked for a long time, starting at about sixteen years old. It seemed like very nearly every boy in my high school class was a cigarette smoker. I was smoking unfiltered cigarettes, as was common in those days, about half a pack a day. It was very much the thing to do.

It was difficult to start. I remember it well. My father had a philosophy that if you are determined to smoke, don't sneak around—do it at home.

My father smoked. As I recall, he smoked Lucky Strikes and Chesterfield cigarettes, which were popular brands in those days. I remember I was in my bedroom listening to the radio and reading a magazine and having a cigarette, and I was eating some French bread, and it made me very sick. I had to go to the bathroom and throw up, and my father laughed because he thought that would teach me not to smoke.

The whole thing made me very ill. In fact, I got sick two or three times. But because of peer pressure in high school to smoke and to drink beer—in those days there was no temptation towards marijuana or anything—I kept trying to get used to smoking, and eventually I did. It took me two or three weeks, maybe even two months—not trying it every day, just on occasion—until I got accustomed to smoking.

Later I switched brands to a filtered brand, Kent, after high school when I went in the Navy in the early fifties. I smoked about a pack a day. All of the years that I smoked cigarettes, I found that I could never smoke more than a pack a day. In the late afternoons and evenings they did not taste good. They left a foul taste in my mouth, and anticipating the cigarette was better than the reality.

In the mid-seventies I quit cigarettes, and to this day I don't know why. I just threw a pack away one day and decided I was not going to smoke again. I took up smoking a pipe. I started smoking about three pipes a day. Eventually, I was smoking five or six pipes a day. I had a pipe in my mouth almost constantly, whether it was lit or not. I had some colleagues and friends who also smoked pipes, and it was something to do together.

Some of my friends who smoked pipes later quit smoking the pipes and took to cigarettes. I found that if I was around them and I didn't have my pipe with me, I would borrow one of their cigarettes. I would tell myself, "Well, one cigarette is not going to get me back to smoking cigarettes," but of course, it did!

So from the mid-seventies until 1983, I was smoking

both cigarettes and a pipe. By 1983 I was smoking about a half a pack of Marlboros a day. I wasn't fooling around with low-tar and -nicotine cigarettes, and since I didn't allow smoking in my office, I would take cigarette breaks in other smokers' offices. I smoked in the evening and on my way to work. I smoked half a pack of cigarettes a day, and my pipe about twice a day, until I had my heart attack. In fact, that very day I remember having some cigarettes and thinking they tasted particularly bad. But right up to the day that I had the heart attack, I was a smoker.

After I quit, I wanted to talk to my wife, Mary Jane, about her smoking and her health. She got angry at me and didn't want to talk about it. She already knew that she shouldn't smoke, but the time had to be right for her to quit. She had my sympathy, because she was trying, but she had smoked since she was a teen-ager and smoked heavily—at least two packs of Marlboros a day.

One day, after she attended Smokenders without telling me, I realized that she hadn't had a cigarette all day. She didn't want other people to know because she was afraid of failing, but she was trying to quit. It was hard for her to get through that first week, but now she is very proud of the fact that she hasn't smoked in more than a year.

Before that she had tried hypnosis. She didn't even want me around when she was listening to the audio tapes on how to quit! She had heard a lot of people say, "Well, I quit for six months," and it was discouraging for her. She was afraid that if she quit and then started again she might never be able to quit permanently.

She was also concerned that if she quit smoking she would gain weight—and she did. She now plans to get into a diet program to lose the weight. She had to lick the smoking problem first, and she did. She's sure she will never smoke again.

For me, the temptation to smoke is completely gone. I just don't like the smell of cigarette smoke. It seems like a dirty habit. Occasionally, and this may sound crazy, but occasionally, on a winter evening, I will get the urge to smoke my pipe. A pipe is something of an evening, indoor activity. Or I'll smell pipe smoke, and that will remind me how enjoyable it was. (Actually, though, it smells better than it tastes, as most pipe smokers would agree.) But it isn't a serious urge; it's not going to turn me back into a smoker. I can pass a pipe shop and say, "Gee, it's like cookies baking, but I am not going to have one." It's pure nostalgia.

It took me about one year or, at most, a year and a half to really dislike smoking. Some people have asked me, "Why didn't you quit sooner? The information was out there about how bad it was for your health." Well, tobacco is like a drug. I had started smoking at a time when you went to the movies and you saw Humphrey Bogart smoking, and it was a very manly thing to do—very macho to have a cigarette dangling from your lip. There was a popular fantasy that the girls thought you were that much more masculine if you had a cigarette after sex.

No one ever said how harmful it was the first ten or fifteen years I was smoking. No one except my mother, who would say, "Why are you doing that? It is going to stunt your growth." But I looked around and I didn't see only short people walking around smoking, so I thought that was all a bunch of baloney that mothers would tell their children to scare them.

Years ago, athletes advertised cigarettes and doctors smoked. I collect old *Life* magazines. I have seen ads in some of them that say, "Doctors who smoke recommend Chesterfield cigarettes." How terrible that in the late thirties *doctors* were recommending brands of cigarettes! That just shows how common smoking was. I mention this only because cigarettes really hooked me. My first fifteen years of smoking, the thing to do was to have a good American breakfast of bacon and eggs and white toast with butter and maybe some coffee, and then to finish that off with a couple of cigarettes. You know what? That's the recipe for a heart attack.

JONI L.
An Ad on TV Convinced

Joni L. was in her early twenties when her parents died. Both had been smokers, and both died of cancer. After she went through a sizable inheritance, she had to make drastic changes to put her life in order. For the past twenty years Joni, now in her early fifties, has worked as a legal secretary and a paralegal, specializing in litigation.

Both my father and mother were smokers. My father had always been a smoker, but not my mother. My mother told me that she had smoked as a teen-ager before I was born. When she found out she was pregnant with me, she stopped smoking. She started again when I was in high school. I am afraid that I may have triggered that, because when she found out that I was smoking on the side in high school, she said, "Well, I used to smoke."

"Oh, Mother, you never did."

"Oh, yes, I did."

"Did you inhale?"

"Yes."

"Show me," I said.

And she did. And that triggered her desire to smoke again after all those years. I guess she thought that if I, her child, was smoking, why couldn't she? She smoked from that day on until she died of cancer. I have carried a terrible guilt all these years as I think I may have been responsible for my mother starting to smoke again.

I remember the way I began to think about smoking. I was about five years old and I was riding my tricycle out in front of the house with a neighborhood playmate. We were talking about what grown-ups did: getting married, having children, drinking, and smoking. I remember saying, "Well, I don't want to get married, I don't want to have children, I'll never drink, but I will smoke." I made a conscious decision for what was, to my child's mind, sophistication. Most adults smoked and I figured it must be fun. I followed my father's example.

When I was about eleven, I got into my dad's cigarettes, stole some matches, and, with my little girlfriend, hid in the weeds of a vacant lot not far from my home. We figured if we hunched down we could smoke and nobody would see us. We didn't realize that the smoke was circling over our heads. I didn't like it: It tasted awful.

I didn't smoke again until I was seventeen. I was a senior in high school, and all of my friends were smoking because it proved you were very grown up, very sophisticated, very much accepted by your peers. Peer pressure and the desire for sophistication and social acceptance triggered my smoking. Still, I had known from the time I was five that I would probably smoke someday.

I was never a heavy smoker. In high school it amounted mostly to going out to the cars in the school parking lot at lunchtime. A group of girls would take their lunches, go out to somebody's car, pile in, laugh and giggle and talk about boys, smoke a couple of cigarettes, and then go back to class. I have never smoked more than a pack a day, very often only three-quarters of a pack a day.

I realize now that I never really liked the taste of cigarettes. I couldn't smoke without having just drunk something or eaten something. If I was under stress and wanted a cigarette to relieve the stress, I would very often have to eat something before smoking. Eating and smoking went hand in hand. I was not a person who could smoke alone. I never got up and smoked first thing in the morning, never smoked last thing before I went to bed. I was never a *heavy* smoker, but I was a *chronic* smoker for nearly eighteen years.

The years 1957 and 1958 were extremely stressful for me. My mother passed away of cancer in the latter part of 1957, I divorced my husband, and in the early part of 1958 my father also died of cancer. In less than fourteen months I had three major traumas. It was a very, very difficult time.

In the 1960s, having gone through most of a large inheritance, I ended up having to sell my home in Menlo Park. It was an extremely difficult period because I was not used to being poor, I was trying to break into the business world in Los Angeles, and I had no connections. I was not smoking any more heavily than before, but still I was smoking, and the stress was mounting.

Then I saw an advertisement on television and it was the actor who played the district attorney on the old "Perry Mason" television program, William Talman. I believe he made the commercial for the American Cancer Society. He was dying of cancer, and he made some television advertisements against smoking which showed him as he appeared on the "Perry Mason" show when he was in good health, and then the camera panned back to him as he looked dying of cancer: emaciated and obviously close to death. His message was, "If you don't smoke, don't start, and if you have started, quit."

That actor reminded me very much of my father. I had lost my father from cancer, my mother from cancer, and now here was this actor in my living room on my television screen telling me why I should stop smoking. He reminded me so much of my father: It was the perfect message for me.

I thought about it for a couple of weeks. I could not shake the memory of that man, that wonderful actor. His face was constantly before me, even while I was at work. Finally I reached the decision to quit. I quit cold turkey after eighteen years.

My method was probably unique to me. I had never heard of anything like it before: I call it the sleep method. I decided to take three days off and do nothing but sleep, which for me was sleeping, getting up, eating, going back to bed, and going to sleep again. I repeated this cycle each day. I did nothing else, had no stress; I just rested and slept. On the fourth day I got up and went to work. I must have read somewhere or heard that by the third or fourth day your body is relieved of the physical craving and after that you just had to work on the mental aspect of smoking. I felt that if my body wasn't craving cigarettes, surely I could control my mind. From that day in 1969, I never touched a cigarette again. It is twenty years now since I quit, and I'm very glad I did!

To show the resolve I had in quitting smoking, on the fourth day after I had quit I started a new job as a legal secretary in Beverly Hills. I had to sit next to another secretary who smoked at her desk. I was surrounded by cigarette smoke, but I never wavered, never took another puff from a cigarette.

Now I cannot be around smokers and I cannot be in a

room full of cigarette smoke. I have developed an allergy to it. I can't breathe, and I get very ill. I feel I owe all this to William Talman and the commercial he did against smoking. He was the one who brought the connection between smoking and cancer into sharp focus for me. I thank God for the new laws prohibiting smoking in the workplace because I have not been able to work in some law firms since I refuse to work around smokers now.

PATRICK REYNOLDS
Committed to Help Others

Patrick, thirty-nine, is the grandson of the founder of the R. J. Reynolds Tobacco Company, one of the largest tobacco companies in the world. As a boy, he watched his father, a heavy smoker, die a slow death from emphysema. In spite of that experience, Patrick started smoking himself. It took him ten years to kick the habit successfully. Today he has invested his inheritance from the R. J. Reynolds fortune in a program to help people quit smoking.

My grandfather, R. J. Reynolds, chewed tobacco and died of cancer of the pancreas. My father smoked heavily and he died at fifty-eight after years of suffering from emphysema. My father's sister, Nancy, smoked, and she also died of emphysema. His other sister smoked and died of cancer. One of Nancy's children, my cousin, smoked, and died recently of cancer. My mother smoked, and I believe that smoking contributed to her death as well.

95

I started smoking at seventeen, sneaking smokes in the basement at Hotchkiss, the prep school where I boarded. I would sneak down to the basement to have one little cigarette once or twice a week from a stale pack of cigarettes. It was very unpleasant initially. Nobody ever inhaled their first few cigarettes without coughing, including me.

I started smoking mostly because it was against the school rules. In fact, smoking was grounds for expulsion. It was an act of pure adolescent defiance. Cigarettes were a way of breaking the rules, and breaking the rules felt great. It was my way of expressing my anger against the school, against authority, against having to take on adult responsibilities. I was really angry about being locked up in boarding school, in classes wearing a coat and tie six days a week.

Occasionally I would smoke in my room. That required elaborate preparations. I put a towel in the crack under the door to keep the smoke from escaping. I would crack the window in such a way that the smoke would flow out the top of the window and the fresh air would flow in the bottom. I'd blow the smoke out the top crack. I had room deodorizer, mouthwash, special soap, cologne to throw around the room and douse my hands in, everything at the ready, in case there was a knock at the door. I thought it all worked because I never got caught, but I found out later that one of the masters at school did see smoke coming out of my room one day and decided not to report me.

As far as I knew, none of my friends smoked because it

wasn't something I did with friends. I did it alone. It was my own personal, private rebellion. I couldn't imagine expressing my anger to adults directly, so I turned the anger inward and did something self-destructive— smoked—instead. All I accomplished was hurting myself. Sixteen or seventeen is a difficult period in life, and that's why so many people are vulnerable to starting smoking at that age.

Once I got to college in California, I was hooked. I smoked a pack a day, and it made me feel older and more confident. It seemed grown-up and sophisticated to smoke. By comparison with all the drugs and craziness that were going on at Berkeley in 1967, smoking was one of the milder forms of rebellion. The peer pressure there was to smoke marijuana.

Cigarettes are a good anxiety-reducer. And once I got accustomed to it, I liked the taste of tobacco. The deep inhaling, deep breathing, is an ancient yoga practice for inducing a calm, meditative state, and smoking helped calm me. Plus, I was a Reynolds; let's not overlook that. The family had helped popularize cigarettes, so there was a certain amount of pride in lighting up a Winston. I always smoked the family products.

I wanted to stop smoking within a year of starting, but I didn't start trying to quit for several years. I tried hypnosis, but I was too uptight to allow myself to let go enough for it to be an effective therapy for me. I really believed that I was so strongly addicted that I couldn't let go of that idea even under hypnosis.

Then I tried Smokenders, which was a system of cutting down on smoking. You start by marking a cigarette to smoke only part of it. I think that takes more willpower and strength than quitting cold turkey. It didn't work because every time you put a cigarette in your mouth you are restimulating the habit and your enjoyment of it. Every time I got to have a cigarette, even when I was down to four or five cigarettes a day, it was very upsetting because I was only going to get that one more cigarette that day, and oh, my *God* . . . So Smokenders didn't work. It might work for someone else, but it didn't work for me.

I tried going cold turkey on my own a few times. I'd make it for a couple of weeks, but it was a very hairy, difficult experience. I was crabby to my friends, I was nervous, I bit my fingernails. The feeling deep inside that I really, really *wanted* a cigarette remained. So that didn't work.

I even tried acupuncture, but I thought the acupuncture was going to make it easy, that it was going to do it for me. It helped a little bit, but it wasn't enough by itself, so I failed. I hadn't really prepared myself to fight the battle of withdrawal. Maybe if I'd tried the acupuncture in conjunction with a strong commitment to being a non-smoker it would have worked. But I didn't, and it didn't.

The best program I tried was Schick. Of all the methods I tried, it was the most effective one, but in the end, it didn't work either. J. Patrick Frawley was the chairman, and we talked, and he loaded me up with materials about addiction, books to read, videos, everything.

The program takes a week. They give you a mild elec-

troshock every time you take a puff in order to give yourself negative reinforcement to counter the positive reinforcement you get from the pleasure of smoking. Now if
each cigarette takes fifteen puffs, and you smoke twenty
cigarettes a day, twenty times fifteen, you get a lot of
positive reinforcement for your habit. Multiply that by
the number of days or weeks or years you've smoked,
and your unconscious mind has hundreds of thousands
of positive associations with smoking. You can make a
conscious decision to quit smoking, but your conscious
mind and unconscious mind don't necessarily work together. All your unconscious mind knows is that smoking
feels good. What Schick does is help deprogram the unconscious mind.

I had such a strong addiction that I went through the
program five times. I'd last three or four weeks or three
or four months and once I lasted eight months, but then
I'd start smoking again. They held follow-up seminars
after the program, but they were really boring. I didn't
like getting in the car, driving to a meeting, and sitting
around listening to people talk about how badly they
wanted a cigarette. I knew that already, and I didn't want
to burn up two hours of my life sitting around listening
to it.

I smoked from 1967 to 1984. That's seventeen years,
but I had periods of non-smoking during that time that
cut the number of years I actually smoked regularly to
more like ten. The thing that would trigger the relapses
was always stress, whether it was positive or negative. I'd
have an argument with my ex-wife, and I'd take out my

anger at her by having a cigarette. Or a lonely moment. Or a sad moment. Positive stress had the same effect. The hardest times for me even now are when I'm relaxed, say, on vacation at a friend's estate. I've had a beautiful meal, we're having an espresso, a friend lights up a cigarette, and I really, *really* want one. It's as though everything is perfect except that one thing is missing: *my* cigarette. Before, I didn't realize that all it takes to get me hooked again is one cigarette. Now I've learned to recognize the danger in these moments, so I'm very wary and careful. I tell myself, "Take it easy, the desire will be gone in five minutes, so just wait it out." I make a conscious decision not to have a cigarette at that tempting moment. I haven't smoked for four years, and now those moments occur much less often.

The thing that finally worked was to quit by myself with an assist from a behavior modification program that I got from a psychologist. When I put together the Reynolds Stop Smoking Program, that was the technique we used. Research done on corporations that support programs to help employees stop smoking finds that smokers do best quitting on their own or with minimal intervention programs, like cassette tapes. They do much better than those in group programs. Only a very small percentage of those in group seminars quit successfully. I invested the money I inherited from my grandfather's fortune into this corporation. I hope I can help undo some of the damage that's been done by tobacco, or at the very least discourage young people from ever starting to smoke.

MICHAEL G.
I Got Tired of the Rigmarole

Michael G. has a Ph.D. in ethnographic history, but has changed careers to become a broker, contracting computer experts to companies. Married for twenty-five years, he is the father of a five-year-old daughter.

I've not smoked for twenty years. I was twenty-five when I quit, and I had smoked for ten or eleven years. I started when I was about fourteen or fifteen, back in prep school in a small town just north of New York City. It started as a game but, sooner or later, everybody got hooked. My father was a very heavy smoker. I ended up smoking Lucky Strike unfiltered cigarettes. I smoked about half a pack a day during high school, close to a pack a day in college and at the Lutheran seminary where I went after college.

After I graduated from the seminary and had already been accepted at graduate school, I worked in a warehouse to earn some money for graduate school and my wedding. There was a lot of dust and gas-driven forklifts, which probably didn't improve the quality of the air (these were pre-EPA days), and I happened to work a forklift a fair amount of the time.

I usually worked lots of overtime because that was the only way you made money in those days. I'd often work over sixty hours a week. I remember this one gray day, the sun was just breaking through the clouds and the breakfast truck had come around for the mid-morning snack, that usual awful sugary kind of food. . . . Anyway, I bought a doughnut and had it with my coffee.

That morning I lit up a cigarette and said, "Hey, I don't like this any more." I put out the cigarette and looked at the cigarette machine: Cigarettes were getting expensive. Now they were forty, maybe forty-five cents a pack, and that had been bothering me. When I was younger I could get cigarettes for as little as twenty-three cents a pack.

Something else was bothering me: Besides carrying around cigarettes in your pocket, you either have to carry enough matches to pass as a pyromaniac, or you carry lighters. And lighters take fluid and flints and you are always diddling around with them.

At least the logistics of smoking cigarettes were not as complicated as the logistics of smoking a pipe, which I had also tried. Smoking a pipe was too much of a pain. I didn't want to carry around a small brain surgery kit just to smoke a pipe for five minutes. I tried cigars and found they didn't taste very good. I even tried a hookah, a bubble pipe, once.

But, back to that morning at the warehouse. . . . I had half a pack of cigarettes with me. That pack stayed in my pocket that whole afternoon. In the evening I threw the pack out on a card table in my bedroom, asked my brother-in-law, "Do you want some cigarettes? Do you want a lighter?" and gave him the cigarettes and the

lighter. About two nights later I had one filter cigarette at a party and it didn't taste very good. I was just
plain getting tired of smoking. That was the last time I
smoked . . . that's about twenty years ago.

You can say that I quit out of sheer laziness. I didn't
want my life to revolve around cigarettes, I didn't want to
have to worry about the change in my pocket, or running
out on holidays, or stuffing a lighter, or carrying all of
this stuff around. Not smoking made life so much simpler! I gained back my shirt pockets, and my pants pockets no longer had long holes torn in them. Suddenly I
didn't have to worry about running out of cigarettes. I
had had this constant worry about supply and logistics. I
came to the conclusion that if I wasn't enjoying it, quit.
The money arguments didn't work, the cancer arguments didn't work, the fitness and health argument
sounded too much like a Southern Baptist summer camp
(they are probably very nice people, but . . .); in the end
smoking was too complicated and too time consuming. I
had to think about too many things to smoke, and I had
plenty of other things I wanted to think about.

This crazy thing of logistics is what really bothered me.
Sometimes you put a pack in your back pocket and sit
down and *crunch*! Or you have tobacco on your lips, and
straight raw tobacco, no matter what the quality, doesn't
taste very good. The nicotine burns. Then there is the
mess, the ashes, what you do with the cigarette if you
want to do something else with your hands. . . .

I still like to play with my hands, but now I do it with
computer keyboards or telephone keyboards, or I'll read

and flip through the pages of computer magazines or journals. There is more than enough to keep one's hands busy; that's never a problem.

CHRIS J.
I Don't Like Feeling Out of Breath

Chris J., thirty-five years old, is a social psychologist evaluating how various groups and organizations promote good health in the community. She was born in England and brought up in the United States. During her childhood her family moved frequently; Chris attended more than twenty schools, most of them in Southern California. Her smoking "career" lasted almost ten years, but it began at age thirteen.

I stopped smoking when I was twenty-two. What happened was that the things you think of as the rewards of smoking when you are young simply aren't there anymore when you become an adult. I mean, you find that smoking is commonplace, and if you are in it for the sophisticated image, that image fades away. And by then, if you're lucky, your sense of self is better developed. Other things are more rewarding as an adult—like your schoolwork, physical activity, and social interactions—so that smoking becomes unimportant to you. Then all you're stuck with at that point is the physiologic component—the addiction—and the smell.

I remember being bothered by having my clothing smell like tobacco, and the fact that people could tell I smoked when I walked into a room even if I wasn't holding a cigarette. In college I supported myself by working in a bank part time. I couldn't smoke on the job. If I wanted to have a cigarette, I had to get up and leave. It got to be a real hassle to have a cigarette.

I started smoking at the end of elementary school, when I was about thirteen. I had a strong interest in horseback riding. A friend and I used to ride horses together after school; we actually trained horses. Her father smoked. He was a farmer from South Dakota, and he smoked unfiltered Camel cigarettes. He also rolled his own cigarettes. She and I used to go home after school and change our clothes and then go out to the stables. Occasionally, she would show up with a pack of cigarettes. I remember walking out to the horses; it was just a ten- or fifteen-minute walk, but it was long enough . . . that is where it all began. She would try smoking—I wouldn't have called it peer pressure then, though I might call it that now. At the time it was just that she was smoking, why wasn't I smoking?

She was my age; we were only two weeks apart. There was something else going on—there was an older girl, probably fifteen or sixteen, who was much more sophisticated than we were, and we looked up to her. She was in high school, and she was someone who did her hair and dressed well, and *she* smoked. She owned one of the horses that we trained, and we wanted very much to be like her. Looking back, I think she was influential in making us want to smoke and be sophisticated in the way that we thought she was.

I remember a few things that I liked about smoking. It was all very image related; one part was the sophistication, and the other was the packaging. I don't know if there is a gender difference here or not, but I think—and this is a terrible stereotype—that women like little things in cute packages. I think this is true for a lot of women, and I remember there was something very attractive about going and buying these little packs of cigarettes. The other thing was the cost—a pack of cigarettes then used to cost around thirty-five or forty cents, which was affordable even for an elementary or high school student. You could get a lot of sophistication and image building for a very small amount of money.

It was easy to buy cigarettes from small liquor stores and gas stations, even though we were obviously too young to buy them legally. It was more difficult and much less likely that we would try to buy them from a large grocery store, like a Safeway.

One day my mother came to me. I can remember the time of day and where I was in the house and all that. It was evident that I had been smoking because I smelled like a cigarette, and she said, "If you do nothing else for me in terms of the way you dress and the way you behave as an adolescent, please don't smoke." She was very sincere, pleading with me not to smoke. I think that probably planted a seed in my mind; it made me think about wanting to quit. I thought, "Boy, she really means this. I probably shouldn't smoke." There was probably a rebellion/defiance component to my smoking, since it was something my parents didn't want me to do.

Neither of my parents ever smoked, and never have. I attribute the ease with which I was able to quit smoking later to that. It seemed natural to me that I shouldn't smoke, and that the whole time I was smoking I probably shouldn't have been smoking.

When I was eighteen I went to England. It was fun to smoke there because English cigarettes are very different—they are smaller and they taste different. American cigarettes are stronger. We used to exchange cigarettes and talk about different brands. At that point, it was still enjoyable to smoke.

Smoking was much more socially acceptable in England than in the United States. Everybody smoked. At that time I smoked about a pack a day, ranging between, say, fifteen cigarettes a day and a pack and a half.

In the beginning, I didn't like smoking: I was trying to start with Camel unfiltered cigarettes, which were just awful. I can't even describe it. To this day, fifteen to twenty years later, I remember how terrible it was. Then, our sophisticated high school friend said, "Well, try these." They were Larks. I don't think Larks are a cigarette anymore, but I remember the purple package with the gold or white labeling. They were very mild cigarettes, but they still weren't mild enough for me. I remember searching for the mildest cigarette I could find. I switched to Tarrytons, which were low tar, low nicotine.

My friend branched off into Marlboros and other very

strong cigarettes. To this day, she still smokes Marl-boros. I couldn't go that way; physiologically, I didn't like it. In the early days, I felt nauseated when I smoked, light-headed and dizzy. I just did not feel good.

I was a true smoker by the time I was fifteen, and I smoked all the way through age twenty-one, or twenty-two, so it was six or seven years. I smoked Lark cigarettes or something equivalent to them in terms of the strength of the tobacco.

Throughout elementary and high school I was very athletic—riding horses, playing softball, running, that sort of thing. I actually ended up buying my own horse in high school, and I did a lot of riding. But when I moved to San Diego to go to college I left the horse behind. I found myself in a new situation—living in the dorms—and smoking was still very acceptable. That's when you start drinking if you're inclined, and I did, so there was a lot of going out to places where smoking and drinking were important focuses. My exercise and physical activity sort of fell by the wayside during the first few years in college.

It was when I began to miss physical activity that I started on the road towards quitting smoking, because I thought, "Well, gee, I want to start exercising again." I could tell I was getting out of shape, and I missed being in shape. I got a bike for my birthday—actually, I got two bikes, one from my boyfriend and one from my parents because they all knew I wanted to get back into physical activity. That was my twenty-first birthday.

I started cycling again. San Diego is a great place to

cycle. I lived in Point Loma, which is a very hilly area, at the midpoint on a very steep hill. One day I went out on my bike with one of my college roommates and started to head up the hill. I realized that I was having a difficult time breathing, and I didn't attribute it all to the hill: I attributed it to my smoking.

From the time I went to San Diego until getting on this bike, there had been two years that I had been physically inactive and smoking at an increased rate. I attributed feeling out of shape and having a hard time breathing not so much to not exercising but to smoking. I thought, "I don't like feeling like an old person. I don't like feeling out of breath." It was a steep hill, but nevertheless for someone who was twenty-one years old, it was very telling. I remember standing on the top of the hill and looking at my roommate and saying, "It's just not worth it. You know, smoking is a bad thing." And that was it. That was the last time I smoked.

I think there were several things that led up to my quitting, but that was the final thing, the most significant thing. I had tried to stop before that, but I can't remember giving it a really hard try. I'd stop for one week or two weeks, just putting the cigarettes aside, and trying not to pick them up again. When I finally decided that there was a good reason to quit smoking, it seemed easy.

I never thought too much about things like cancer. I was too young at the time I quit to worry about that sort of thing. It was very much oxygen related, something that is important if you exercise a lot. Even now when I am feeling lazy and say, "I don't want to get out on my bike," I think about the air, about how good it feels to get plenty of oxygen into your brain after sitting in an office all day, and that is enough incentive to get me out. I was used to the high that exercise gives, so it's a good incentive for me.

Now looking back, I do remember a pain in my lungs that I had not felt before—a raspy feeling. When I heard friends who coughed a lot in the morning from smoking I thought, "Am I going to be that way in a few years?" I didn't think about cancer or heart disease, I am sure I didn't think about chronic disease, but I did think about clogging up my breathing system and being less physically capable of exercising.

The interesting thing is that I had a roommate who smoked and I had a boyfriend who smoked, and that was a problem with the boyfriend. It began to bother me. I think you have to go one way or another—either other people's smoking bothers you or you start smoking again. It's hard to stay neutral about having close friends who smoke when you don't.

When I go to hotels I always request non-smoking rooms now. In restaurants and on airplanes I request the non-smoking section. If I am in a non-smoking section and someone is smoking, I'll ask them to put their cigarette out. A neighbor came over and wanted to give me some little housewarming gifts, and she asked if she could come in. I said, "Yes, you can, but your cigarette has to stay outside."

I live alone now, but I wouldn't date or get into a relationship with someone who smoked. Wouldn't it be awful to meet a terrific person who smoked? That would be tough.

BOB L.
My Wife and I Quit the Same Day

Bob L., forty-nine, has worked a granite rock quarry for twenty-three years, first as a heavy equipment operator and then as supervisor of rock crushing. Bob and his wife have three grown children, with children of their own. On weekends, he and his wife take off in their motor home. They both enjoy fishing.

About three years ago I quit smoking for the last time, because of my wife. Smoking was starting to bother her health—she was coughing a lot. She said, "Honey, I'm going to stop smoking." And I said, "Well, honey, if you're going to quit, then I'm going to quit, too." She smoked about three packs a day, the same kind of cigarettes I did. I thought, "If she is going to quit, it would be a lot easier for her and me to quit together." We both quit on the same day, the same week.

If it weren't for her health, I probably would still be smoking because it didn't bother my system. I know it really bothers a lot of people. But I have to say honestly that it never bothered me. But it made my wife cough a lot and get real deep chest pains. And, no joking, money was a big factor. We figured it up one time and it cost $1,100 a year for her and me to smoke. That played some part in deciding to quit, but the biggest part was the health factor.

I still craved cigarettes for some time after I quit. I had to have the willpower to say, "No, I am not going to take one." Your body does crave those cigarettes for quite a while—like maybe three, four, or five months. I think the key to quitting smoking is yourself: I don't think anybody can tell somebody to quit; it has to be your own decision. Once you make up your mind, you can quit. I don't think you can go to a hypnotist or to a school. I think it is all up to the individual. A lot of people say they can't quit, but down deep, I don't think they want to quit. They really want to smoke. They say, "How did you do it? I just can't quit smoking." Well, you *can* quit, because the day you say, "That's it. I am not going to smoke," you can flat out quit.

Since I quit, I eat a little more. Food tastes a lot better, and with the food tasting better, instead of grabbing a cigarette, we tend to eat more. My wife has gained weight since we've quit smoking.

I can honestly say that quitting did make me a little bit nervous in the beginning. I got tense because sometimes my subconscious mind was saying, "I want a cigarette," and then my conscious mind would say, "No, you're not going to have a cigarette," so I had a tug-of-war between my subconscious mind and my real mind.

I remember how my dad smoked until he was about forty-five, and one day he quit. He just threw his cigarettes out the window, and that was the last time he smoked. He just flat quit, and that was it.

I started smoking young, probably fourteen years old, about 1952. I think one of the reasons I started is that all the other kids were doing it, so it was something like, "The other kids do it, so why not me?" I think it's the same with drugs and everything else.

In the beginning my body tried to reject the nicotine. But I told myself, "I'm going to make myself smoke," because everybody else was doing it, and I thought it was kind of a smart thing. Pretty soon your body builds up a tolerance to it, and you're hooked. I would say it took my body a couple of months to get hooked on it.

I used to smoke about two, two and a half packs a day. I usually smoked filter cigarettes—Virginia Slims. My wife did, too. We both smoked when we got married; I was nineteen and she was seventeen. I smoked two and a half packs a day for thirty-three years.

I had quit once before, about ten years ago. At that time I decided to quit because it interfered with my work. I was always grabbing a cigarette, trying to smoke it while I was working, and it got in the way. I got mad at myself for smoking and just threw the things away and said I wasn't going to smoke no more. When you're trying to do something and you have a cigarette in your mouth and the smoke is in your eyes and your eyes are watering, you just get mad. I said, "That's it, I am not smoking no more."

I didn't smoke for a year. Then I started again. The reason is that a lot of times you're sitting around with the guys and having a beer or something, and the next thing you know, "Well, I'm going to have me a cigarette." So

I'd have a cigarette, and the first one made me dizzy. It took a little while to get used to it again. That dizzy spell is your body trying to reject the nicotine, but pretty soon I was smoking again anyway.

When other people smoke it doesn't bother me a bit. As a matter of fact, I can smell their smoke, and I don't even crave one. But for the first few weeks, whenever I smelled a cigarette, I had to have some willpower not to ask for one. I really had to watch myself, but once I got over that hump it was fine.

I am happy I have quit, you bet. I'll never, ever start back again. My wife either. We will never, ever go back to smoking again. Now my house is clean. Oh, it used to smell of smoke. We had to wash the walls down. When you're smoking like that you don't know how dirty the house gets from just nicotine and smoke. It's unbelievable.

LOUISE G.
The Change in Public Attitude
Has Helped Me

Louise G., sixty-three, and the mother of five children, practiced law for seventeen years before retiring to devote her considerable energy to tennis, bridge, and Scrabble. She lives in a turn-of-the-century house in a quiet town south of San Francisco. Her smoking led to the trauma of a bad fall.

I had a weight problem when I was young, and smoking changed my metabolism so that I could eat as much as I wanted without gaining weight. I started smoking when I was sixteen. My brother and I would sneak into the bathroom with a pack of Camels and smoke. I enjoyed it right away. I was a senior in high school then, and by the summer between high school and college, I was smoking a pack a day.

I always smoked a pack a day. I smoked all through college. I smoked through my four pregnancies and five children. Nothing could convince me to stop smoking.

Every one of my children objected to my smoking—loudly and often. They left no doubt as to the intensity of their disapproval. Worse, they set me a good example: Not one of them ever smoked. Even worse were my four grandchildren, who begged me to stop smoking practically from the time they could talk. But none of this inspired me to stop. I didn't have a cough. I had no trouble breathing. And I liked smoking.

Two of my daughters are nurses, and they, of course, were the most outspoken of my children about how bad smoking was for my health. They would say, "We'll take you to the hospital and make you look at the emphysema patients. *That* will convince you to quit." The idea that someday I might not be able to breathe was very frightening, but even that didn't work. Nothing worked.

There were some things I just couldn't do without a cigarette. Ironing was one, sewing was another. When I was working with my hands I liked to have a cigarette going at the same time. I would stop smoking when I had a cold. I had one fairly serious illness when I was in my early thirties, and for a long time I couldn't smoke. Well, I could hardly wait until I could start smoking again. I really looked forward to it, as that was the only way I enjoyed doing things like sewing: Sewing and cigarettes always went together for me.

I used smoking as a pleasant way to break up the day. When the mail came, I'd sit down, light a cigarette, and read the mail. Or I'd tell myself, "First I'll have a cigarette, and then I'll do that chore."

There were some problems with smoking. I had an awful tendency to burn holes in my clothes and in the car upholstery. I worried constantly that I'd left a cigarette burning when I left the house, and I'd go back home to reassure myself that I hadn't.

Another problem was that, even when I smoked, I hated the smell of stale cigarette smoke. I remember now how offensive and unpleasant it was to open the door of my car and smell the stale tobacco. I didn't mind having other smokers around me. I played bridge with three other smokers, and the smell was not particularly objectionable. I was so used to the odor of cigarette smoke that I didn't even notice immediately if a smoker had been in my house. I couldn't smell the smoke on clothes either. It was only the smell of stale smoke that was so terribly unpleasant.

Anyway, not even the offensive smell of stale smoke in the car or the holes I routinely burned in my clothes deterred me from smoking until something happened one morning in the fall of 1983. I will never forget the details of that morning as long as I live.

That morning I got up, went to the bathroom, brushed my teeth—I couldn't stand to smoke until I had brushed my teeth—and then I lit a cigarette. That had been my routine for years. I truly enjoyed that first cigarette; it tasted *so* good.

That morning I lit my first cigarette and after a few puffs I felt terribly sick to my stomach and terribly dizzy. I felt sicker and worse than I ever had in my whole life. I was so dizzy that I fell down, cracking my head on the bathroom floor. You know how you feel when you are afraid you are going to die? That's how I felt. It was awful. My kids took me to the hospital and I realized that I should never smoke again. And I haven't.

That was my last puff, that cigarette in the bathroom. Smoking is permanently intertwined in my mind with that awful fall, that terrifying sick and dizzy sensation. I am sure that it was the cigarette that triggered the sickness, that dizziness and weakness and bad fall. I have a very definite connection in my mind between the cigarette and the fall. That's what has kept me away from cigarettes since that day. I haven't touched one since.

I am fairly sure that if I smoked a cigarette now and didn't get sick that I'd probably be hooked again. I've dreamed that I smoked and wakened not quite sure whether it really happened. That's scary, because I don't ever want to smoke again. I've made a bargain with myself about cigarettes exactly like the one I've made about candy: never again, not even one!

Never again? Well, maybe when I'm eighty I'll have another Hershey bar, but I haven't had one in forty-two years. And sometimes I think that if I make it to ninety-five, and there isn't much I can do with myself anyway, maybe I'll try smoking again. . . .

Could I get hooked again if I tried one cigarette? I think so. The only way I've been able to stay away from cigarettes for the last four years is to know that I can never have another cigarette, not one.

Before my collapse I had tried to cut down on smoking with low-tar cigarettes. I ended up smoking three packs a day instead of one, and not enjoying it. In the last few years before I quit, I'd started asking clients if they minded if I smoked while they were in my office. I guess that was my attempt to integrate myself into the new world, the world where smoking was no longer socially acceptable. There were ten lawyers in my law office, and I was the only one who smoked.

The change in attitude toward smoking from the fifties to today helped me make the connection between smoking and my fall. It's interesting to watch movies of the forties, fifties, and sixties—everyone's smoking! If there had not been so much public information about how bad smoking is for your health, I'd probably have started smoking again the minute I recovered from my fall.

My life changed when I stopped smoking. I gained thirty pounds, most of which I've taken off. I can't eat as much as I used to without gaining weight. It wasn't that I ate more when I quit; it's that the same amount I ate then now makes me put on weight, so I have to eat less and play tennis more. I appreciate the fact that my car doesn't smell of stale tobacco any more, and I don't burn holes in my clothes and the car upholstery any more, and I don't worry about burning the house down any more. These are big differences. As far as my general health goes, I don't believe it's made any difference.

It makes me very sad that my fifteen-year-old grand-daughter has started smoking. I understand smoking has become epidemic among teen-age girls. When she was eight or nine, she used to beg me to stop: "Don't smoke, Granny. I don't want you to die." Her eight-year-old sister wrote an essay in school that said, "This is a description of a happy day. A happy day is one that my sister would stop smoking so her lungs and teeth would not get black and she would not die. I am worried about her smoking. I want her to live to a hundred and two." That story is pasted on our refrigerator, but I'm afraid the fifteen-year-old doesn't pay much attention to it.

JUNE H.
Something Is Different . . .

June H., in her mid-thirties, is a vivacious woman who works in the public relations department of a major corporation. As a single parent, she has two daughters. Recently she moved to a quiet suburb outside the city and is looking forward to going back to school. After many efforts to quit, she says she doesn't care about smoking anymore.

I was pregnant in 1980 with my second daughter, and during that whole pregnancy my doctor kept saying, "June, the baby is not growing. You have to quit smoking." And the more she told me, the more I smoked. It was weird. Every Monday I would say, "Okay, this is my last cigarette," but I couldn't quit. I would think, "Oh, no. Something is going to be wrong with my baby," but I'd still have the cigarette.

After the baby was born, every Monday for three years I woke up saying, "I'm not going to smoke anymore." I would make it through the day, but then Monday night I would smoke, and I'd say, "Well, I'll quit next week." And I'd try to quit again the next week. This went on for years.

I started smoking when I was fifteen, in the tenth grade. Everyone else did, and we thought it was in. I got pregnant when I was in the eleventh grade. I was sixteen. I couldn't smoke during that pregnancy—it was a difficult pregnancy—but when my daughter was four months old, I started smoking again.

When you have smoked your whole life, it takes time to change. I tried to quit almost from the beginning. One time I went to a hypnotist and quit smoking for about two days—that was it! I was always a nervous kid, and I always thought that I smoked out of nervousness. That was my release. . . . If something was going wrong, smoking was the way I released all of the tension.

After that I tried to quit many times. When I came to work for this corporation in 1979, they offered the employees a Smokenders program. The company paid for part of the program, and if you still weren't smoking in three months you would get half of your money back. After six months, you would get all of your money back. When I went into this program, I quit smoking for three weeks.

In 1985 I quit for one month, then I started again. In 1986 I quit for about two months on my own. See, I always wanted to quit, but something always came up that made me nervous, and I would smoke again. Either something happened in my family or something happened on the job. I was very nervous, unsettled. I am real hyper, so I used that as an excuse.

In March of 1987, my younger daughter's father, who is a smoker, had one lung collapse, and we went to visit him at the hospital. On the way home I lit up a cigarette, and my youngest girl started crying and said, "Mom, if you don't quit smoking, you are going to die like my father." Her father didn't die, but we had just seen him in the hospital, and he had all of these tubes coming out from his body all over the place.

I felt bad. . . . I put down that cigarette and didn't smoke for about eight weeks. Then I started again. It seemed like I could only make it without smoking for about eight weeks.

In 1987 I went through a period when I started getting chest pains. One night I was smoking a cigarette, and when I inhaled, it felt like a hand had just squeezed my heart. I caved over a little bit, and I thought, "My God, I'm not even thirty-five, and I am going to end up having a heart attack."

And what did I do? I went and smoked three cigarettes in a row. I thought, "Oh, no. I might die of a heart attack." Yet, all of this time, I was just puffing one cigarette after another.

Smoking became an obsession, and it wasn't fair to anyone around me. The whole house, everyone, was complaining about my smoking. It got to the point where the only place I could smoke was in the bathroom. I found myself in the bathroom the majority of the time that I was at home because that was the only place they would let me smoke. Smoking wasn't much fun any more.

I felt sorry for my older daughter because I would give her my cigarettes and say, "Give me two a day," but then I would end up asking her for more. One night I woke her up at one in the morning. I said, "Michelle, where did you put my cigarettes?" because she would hide them. I looked in her closet and her drawers. She said, "Mom, I am not giving you one." I said, "Michelle, either you are going to give me a cigarette, or else I am going to get up and go to the store." She got up, threw my cigarettes at me, and said, "Mom, don't bother me with your not smoking any more."

This time something is different. I have not smoked for over five months. It all started last June. Michelle was going to graduate from high school. Just before she graduated, I started getting headaches from smoking. I would cough every morning and cough up phlegm. I would gag when I brushed my teeth in the morning.

After her graduation party I had a couple of cigarettes,

and all my girlfriends told me, "Well, June, you said when Michelle graduated you would quit smoking." And I said, "I am, I will." Michelle said, "Well, Mom, I graduated, so I guess you have to quit smoking." I said, "I guess I have to."

The next day when I woke up I didn't have any more cigarettes in the house, but there was half a butt in the ashtray and I unrolled it, straightened it out, struck a match and inhaled the smoke. I literally choked on the cigarette and I thought, "What am I doing? Here I go, I am going to kill myself again, I am back to the same old thing. . . ." As soon as I lit the cigarette I started getting my headache again, the same headache I had been getting for a couple of weeks, and I thought, "June, you're going to die with a cigarette in your mouth." And so I crushed that cigarette out that Friday morning and I haven't had one since.

I quit cold turkey. Everything seemed to come together all at once. In March 1987, my younger daughter's father's lung collapsed, and he had to have it removed. That same month, my uncle, also a heavy smoker, died of cancer. In June my older daughter graduated, and I'd sworn for years that I'd quit when she graduated. I'd been smoking a pack a day for twenty years, but I quit cold.

It was hard for the first two months. I was very nervous, and my stomach was upset practically all the time. That had always been more than enough to get me back to smoking in the past, but this time I dealt with the issues. I said, "June, having a cigarette isn't going to make you less nervous. It'll make you more nervous because you'll be smoking again and worrying about coughing up phlegm and cancer and heart attacks again." Every time I felt lousy I told myself it was because my body was getting rid of the poison, getting the nicotine out of my system.

There was one time when if it hadn't been for the worst hurricane in history I would have gone out and bought a pack of cigarettes. That was the last day of my vacation in Jamaica, and Hurricane Gilbert was coming. My friend and I were preparing ourselves for the hurricane to hit. Everything was fine. When we went into our hotel room it started to rain, and I felt this tremendous urge to smoke. If I could have gone to the store, I would have bought some cigarettes, and I would have smoked. And the more it stormed, the more the wind howled, the more I wanted a cigarette.

I thought, "If I am going to die, I might as well smoke." I told my friend, "If I could get a cigarette right now, I would be smoking." "June, don't," he said, "because the hurricane is going to be over, we are going to go back home, and then you are going to regret it."

When I got back home, my kids said, "Mom, we can't believe that you didn't smoke while you were there." Out of my whole vacation that was the only time that the urge came. Other than that, I was swimming every day, and I felt great.

I think I have done it this time. I feel so much better now. My headaches aren't as bad. I have not gagged at all since I quit smoking.

Now that I have not smoked for five months many things are changing. I wear contact lenses, and often when I was smoking my eyes were red and sticky. It seemed like I had to rinse out my contacts a couple of times a day. But now I don't. I put in my lenses in the morning, and they last all day.

Under my eyes my skin used to be so tight, but now it isn't. It feels good. Around my cheekbones, it feels good. In fact, my skin feels cleaner, and it looks cleaner, and the dry feeling it used to have is gone. A lot of people recently have said, "June, what are you doing to your face? It looks so clear." One friend said, "June, you look like you've gotten two years younger." But they didn't know I'd quit smoking, because I'm not going around telling everyone I quit. People say, "God, you look so young since the last time I saw you. What have you done?" And I say, "I don't know, but I think it's because I quit smoking."

Food tastes different too; my whole cooking style is different. I don't put a lot of salt or pepper on my food anymore. I used to dump lots of spices into my food just to be able to taste it, and now I don't. I used to have to have a lot of sweets, but now when I eat a candy bar, I don't like it anymore. I used to eat about three candy bars a day. I could always have a doughnut in the morning, but now I don't want all of that sugar. I don't need it like I used to.

To me, tobacco is worse than heroin. I worked at Stanford University at a drug clinic in 1974, and I saw people who were hooked on heroin, and do you know, I always felt like cigarettes were just as bad because there is a terrible withdrawal. You get depressed when you quit, physically you go through a lot, and you are always thinking about cigarettes. It is an obsession.

Now the only time that I think about cigarettes is at the end of a day, when I say to myself, "June, you are doing great." I tell myself that every day. All my friends who have gone through my millions of assertions, "I'm going to quit this week, I'm going to quit this week," say, "June, I never could believe that you would quit smoking." All of them tell me that. Even my daughters. They say, "Mom, I can't believe you haven't had a cigarette." They can't believe it because they heard me tell them a million times before that I was going to quit.

I don't think I'll smoke again this time. Now I don't care about it. I really don't.

LESLIE M.
Things Smell Good Now

Leslie, thirty-one, is a writer and poet. She has spent all of her adult life in the university world: ten years in undergraduate and graduate studies in creative writing and English and four years as a teacher of creative writing at a small women's college. She is certain that her academic background not only allowed but encouraged her smoking habit for a number of years. Leslie's interview is followed by excerpts from letters she wrote to a close friend soon after she had smoked her last cigarette.

I have been a non-smoker for a hundred and twenty days today—but my eleven years as a chain smoker are still as vivid and sweet to me as youth itself. I have not had so much as a puff of a cigarette since I paid $200 to have myself hypnotized one afternoon last May, but I have watched hungrily as other people smoked around me, and hundreds of moments already I have been on the verge of reaching for someone else's cigarette left burning in an ashtray or waving near my face.

Like most young people of my generation, I was certain the world was a dangerous place and would do me in before I could do myself in with something like cigarettes. My first cigarettes were those we snuck down by the ravine in my subdivision. As a daughter of the white upper middle class, I was terribly interested in passive rebellion, and smoking was one of the most available expressions of that. Of course, those first cigarettes tasted vile, and staggering up out of the ravine, a little dizzy from the experience, my girlfriends and I chewed onion grass to hide the smell on our breath. Between the ages of sixteen and nineteen or twenty, I confined my smoking to parties, bars—situations where alcohol was the primary agent of rebellious behavior—but I was still often repelled by people who chain-smoked in the daytime.

Nineteen seventy-four was my first year in college; I don't know if it was indicative of the times or the place or both, but women there seemed to be taking up smoking in great numbers. My favorite professors, sassy, smart, professional women, held court in tiny offices crammed with impressive-looking books and blue clouds of smoke. It was not unusual for them to smoke during class, gesturing with their cigarettes. It was also not unusual then to find classrooms supplied with stacks of ashtrays. No one asked if anyone minded smoking. All the campus radicals I admired most seemed to chain-smoke. I was trying to make myself into a woman writer, a poet: I had a photograph of Edna St. Vincent Millay holding a cigarette and looking pensive; I saw Jane Fonda play Lillian Hellman in the movie *Julia,* chain-smoking and throwing her typewriter dramatically out of the window. I associated smoking with bluestocking women, independent women who turned their intelligent eyes on men who annoyed them and blew smoke in their faces. I found smoking a very useful deterrent to drunk and potentially pawing fraternity boys, a socially acceptable way of surrounding oneself with boundaries.

Then I fell madly in love with a dangerously handsome man who told me right off that he couldn't stand to see attractive women smoking cigarettes, and I didn't much care because I didn't then feel I *needed* to smoke. But when he suddenly disappeared from my life and couldn't be reached even by phone, I decided to mourn his passing with a bottle of scotch and a chain of Salem Light 100s that lasted a few days, at the end of which I realized I had come to like the taste of cigarettes, scotch or no scotch. And in playing out my agony over the loss of my beautiful boyfriend, I had hung over the typewriter pounding out stories and poems of revenge and made the most powerful association of my life: cigarettes with writing.

Four months after having my last cigarette and it is still difficult to be at the typewriter without a cigarette in the ashtray. I still believe that cigarettes actually helped me think, that they helped me focus and make the connections that I need for effective communication. I liked being a smoker for many years. I liked pictures of myself looking writerly in profile with a cigarette in my hand. I liked the fraternal feelings of hanging out in student lounges and dark pubs with other writers who were chain-smoking, and now I am a little unhappy sometimes that I have to avoid such scenes because they make me too nostalgic for my old smoking self.

Quitting smoking was one of the hardest things I have ever done, so hard, so painful that the strongest deterrent to my taking up smoking again is the thought of ever going through withdrawal again. I began to quit in stages: First I bought a new car and decided I was never going to smoke a cigarette in that car, even though I was—and intended to continue being—a chain smoker then. I did not smoke in that car, and I wouldn't let anyone else smoke in it either, which seemed odd to my many smoker friends, but it was the first of a number of inconveniences I tried to cause myself over smoking. The second step was the loss of my cigarette case, a metal case with an enameled design that I had bought the very month I began smoking full time. I loved that cigarette case; it kept my cigs dry and smooth and found its way back to me on numerous occasions when I had left it at parties or bars. But I lost that case one night about a year before I actually quit smoking. I knew where I had lost it, a little jazz club on the edge of town, but I decided not to call about it the next day. I thought if I had to live with no cigarette case, my cigarettes would get wet and smashed and the inconvenience would eventually convince me I didn't need to smoke any more.

Then I tried a trial run: I went to teach creative writing at a summer school/camp for the arts where I have spent a number of happy summers. I knew that the effects of the altitude would make smoking yet more problematic for me when I first went up, and I knew that being out in the woods it would be inconvenient for me to drive into town to buy cigarettes. I also resolved to buy cigarettes I didn't like so that I would only smoke when I was desperate. This way, with sheer willpower, I managed to get myself down from a pack and a half a day to three cigarettes a day. I thought I would leave the mountains a non-smoker, but I then was scheduled to attend a writers' conference and I was terrifically nervous about that because I was to read my poems to an audience of rather important and intimidating people. On the flight to the conference I opted for the non-smoking section, but the man who met my plane was happily smoking away, and when we arrived at the party of writers in progress at the convention center, all happily yakking away in their clouds of smoke, I greedily smoked a whole pack. I was a hacking, wheezing chain smoker once again.

It was another year before I again decided I needed to

quit smoking. But this time I had clear reasons: I had just passed the age of thirty. I began to feel old, a little dried-up looking. I could see the beginnings of "smoker's face" on me: the sallow skin, the bags around my eyes, the dry cross-hatching. I admit I am vain, and my vanity was much more powerful, finally, in persuading me that smoking was detrimental to me than any of the hundreds of pamphlets and articles on the nasty effects of smoking that my mother sent me regularly in the mail. I looked in the mirror and thought that quitting smoking might be like getting oneself a very expensive facial: my color would improve, my hair would be healthier, my eyes brighter.

I called a hypnotist and made an appointment. I called my mother and told her I was quitting smoking for her Mother's Day present so I couldn't back out. I sat on a bench outside the hypnotist's office and had my last cigarette. I said to myself: This is my last cigarette ever. I took every drag deeply. A few men in business suits passed me on my bench and smiled. I wondered if they suspected that I was a woman smoking the last cigarette of her life. I smoked that cigarette right down to the butt, and then I threw the rest of the pack, lighter and all, in the nearest trash can.

The next three days were a nightmare, and the whole first month of withdrawal was a trial I never wish to repeat. During that month I was trying to write a lot of letters to a very close friend of mine, partly because writing letters helps me keep sane and in control of my feelings and partly because I wanted to keep myself comfortable at the typewriter and try to prevent my decision to quit smoking from affecting my writing.

The excerpts from those letters describe some of the things I worked through as I cast off the most powerful habit of my life. . . .

May 8, 1988

Dear Joanne,

I have actually done it—gone to the hypnotist and gotten the stop smoking routine. I became a non-smoker at 3 P.M. on Friday, and now, about noon on Sunday, I am rather a mess about it. I figure that at a pack a day and about ten minutes per cigarette, I was spending somewhere between three and four hours a day with a cigarette in my hand—times twelve years. No wonder I feel fragmented, confused, unfocused. Writing is very difficult; paying attention to anything for very long is difficult. I began a letter to you yesterday, got about a page written, spaced out, and shut off the power to the computer before I had saved the file, so the whole page I'd written was zapped. I'm not sure that the hypnosis is really the miracle cure they claim it to be. I want a cigarette more than ever, but after I paid two hundred bucks to have someone tell me I don't want a cigarette, I think of all the money down the drain if I do smoke a cigarette.

I get absentminded and find myself going to the drawer where I kept my cigarette supply, or digging in my purse while I am on the phone. I tried chewing gum, but that makes my jaws hurt after a while, and so I went to the grocery this morning and bought a box of wooden toothpicks. I have them here by the typewriter and find that they are the best answer to cigarette cravings. I remember that one of my teachers quit a long smoking habit when I was his student, and we all used to think it was pretty funny how he'd sometimes have two toothpicks hanging on his lip—he had a very hard time quitting smoking—he finally managed it. But I am having trouble hanging onto ideas, trouble sitting here at the computer and having the same sort of concentration I used to have when I did smoke. I wonder if smoking really did help me focus and concentrate or if I only believed that it did. I'm sure the latter. Well, this morning when I got up, I reached into the cupboard for some clothes and noticed the smell in there—the general stale smell of cigarettes—my whole closet reeks—and I never noticed it before. My mother always swore that the suitcases I left at home were full of cigarette smell, and I thought she exaggerated. I spent a good portion of my time yesterday cleaning the nicotine stains off the windows, picture glass, walls, and blinds. That's an activity that always grosses me out because the nicotine is so sticky and yellow and nasty—I figured grossing myself out that way would reinforce my resolve. I notice that even after a day and a half, my own sense of smell is improved many times and the inside of my mouth tastes good—sort of fruity and sweet. I never realized how ugly that taste of cigarettes was in my mouth. My friend Janet told me that when she quit smoking, she was sure that her lips got fuller and the bags under her eyes went away.

Probably the most effective motivation for my decision to quit was the face of a woman. . . . She's a great lady, feisty, older, smart—but her face is positively an example of the smoker's face they show you in those scare tactic programs. It's true that smoking ages the skin in a way nothing else does. Women who have smoked for a long time begin to look like ashtrays themselves. This woman is a prime example. Her skin is wrinkled and gray, and her gums and teeth are yellowish like dog teeth. If you look hard, you see that this woman is neither very old nor naturally very ugly. She also has that thinning, limp smoker's hair and yellowish fingers. I was so frightened of becoming like that that I was motivated to quit. So this is all to say that it's vanity that made me quit—and vanity that will probably keep me a non-smoker.

Janet tells me that when she quit, she cried for two weeks and the horror of the whole experience was enough to keep her from ever smoking again. She's been helping me along—telling me things like how her hair got bright and shiny again after she quit, how her skin plumped up and glowed, and her energy level soared, but she told me as well that I would have to remember that I would always be an ex-smoker, that if I ever even took so much as a puff of a cigarette again, I could ruin all my hard work, trigger the addiction anew. It's all an interesting psychological experiment—the gaps in my experience—all my adult life to have been a smoker. I try to remember it all—it was before I became a writer, before I knew anything about anything. The only time I was a non-smoker was when I was a kid—and then I began smoking, though not chain-smoking, when I was sixteen, and I became a smokestack when I was about nineteen and had gotten very fat from endless dorm food and adolescent depression. The smoking had a great many functions in my life then—it helped me thin down; it was a great social control, a way to keep one's physical distance from a man in a bar or at a fraternity party. One thing I am feeling now that Janet said she felt too—was vulnerability. The habit is some sort of wall between you and the world, and really a weapon too. Blowing smoke in someone's face is a good way to get them to leave you alone. But the whole thing also functions as a psychological wall between the self and the world, and I do feel rather exposed right now, as if I am wearing my heart on my sleeve.

I've been riding my bike a lot these last two days, and when I'm out riding, I don't feel as inclined to want a cigarette. Yesterday I rode to the park and the place where the fountain surrounded by magnolia trees is. There weren't many folks out, so I helped myself to one of those basketball-sized magnolia blossoms, put it in my backpack, and rode on home with it; it's so huge it takes up a whole big serving bowl, and the perfume from it is overwhelming—all through the house I can smell it. Amazing. I don't know if the blossom is really unusually powerful or if my non-smoking status renders my nose so much more capable I can smell anything. I know that riding my bike today was more pleasurable than yesterday because I could smell every flower I passed and often identify it—and while the smells are strong enough for even a smoker to detect, the pleasures are much heightened now. I'm wishing I could have that house full of lilacs before me again—now I could appreciate them all the more.

May 13, 1988

Dear Joanne,

Today marks exactly one week without a cigarette, and though it's a lot better than it was the first three days, I am still missing cigs a lot. The first three days were hell. I was feeling crazy, mean, restless, and had terrific night-mares in which I was smoking like crazy. When I woke up, my chest hurt as if I had been chain-smoking; my throat was sore and I felt positively battered. The next few nights, I couldn't sleep at all. I got up and wandered around the house in the dark sucking on toothpicks and wanting a cigarette so badly I thought I'd get dressed and go out to an all-night store. But I held out. I inspect my face every day now to find the changes—the slow but wonderful changes in my skin and hair. My face is getting softer and the bags under my eyes are actually fading. This is not my imagination. There simply seems to be more moisture under my skin. It looks plump. In order to keep myself from wanting cigs, I've taken endless bike rides and am enjoying the way my lungs feel better and cleaner every day. I can't believe how much more breath I have. When I exert myself, I don't feel that pain in my chest—and there seems to be more room in me for air in general. I've been riding first thing in the morning and just before dark at night—mostly on the park bike path, which is probably a four-mile run if I do full circle. It takes about an hour to do the whole thing and back from my front door. Last night I did it all twice, till my legs ached—and last night was the first night that I actually slept soundly and well since I quit smoking. I am growing to love that park and bike path. It's so amazing both morning and night.

Probably my single greatest benefit in quitting smoking is what I can smell now—since I am a person who responds so much to smell. And since I have ridden that path so many times this week, I've gotten to know which spots will smell what way, and I can anticipate each tree and patch of flowers before I get to it. The other great thing to do on the park trail is check out the joggers. They are almost all men and quite an attractive bunch. I can smell them too when I whiz past on my bike as they huff and puff in the Texas heat. They, of course, have no idea how deeply I am breathing in their intimate smells, and I love the secret feeling of stealing those smells from them. And already I am beginning to get a sense of who the regulars are, who does the loop more than once, and how long it takes each one to get around.

God how I miss smoking. I have a toothpick in my mouth at this very minute. I've become as addicted to them as I ever was to cigarettes, and the toothpick is quite an ugly habit. I look like a real hick. If my mother could see me, I'm sure she'd rather have me smoking.

Last night I went to a small party. On the late end of the party there were a number of people smoking—probably everyone in the room except three of us. Of course, they were all writers. At first I loved the smoke and breathed deeply of it, but after about an hour, it started to smell bad and I got a headache. When I came home I noticed the smell of smoke in my hair and clothes and had to take a shower before bed because it bugged me so much. I thought maybe that was some sort of break-through, a sign that I really am changing my mentality from that of a smoker to that of a non-smoker. I did talk to two other folks last night who had quit long-time smoking habits. One woman told me that she slept differently now, that she dreamed more and slept more soundly since she quit smoking, but also that she went to bed much earlier because there was something about smoking that kept her awake. And it's true I have been dreaming much more and sleeping differently, though at first I had great insomnia, and the dreams are not all that soothing.

Last night I could smell each person I talked to. I could smell the fabric of their clothes and the soap they'd used to shower. If I get close to people's hair, I can smell shampoo and that fur smell that hair has. There's something very sensuous about not smoking. I want to touch everyone, get close, smell skin. I want to put my nose against heads and shoulders and arms. I smell my own skin, my hands and wrists and breasts. It's quite wonderful and sexy. I feel sort of sexually charged by it all and wonder if I haven't been missing out on something all these years.

Of course, bad smells now are exaggerated, too. The fruit stand next door has begun to stink. They throw the rotting stuff out back and it continues to rot in the sun. My neighbor and I are worried about it because the smell drifts in our windows when the wind is going a certain direction—and the loose rotting produce has drawn some monster city rats. I haven't seen them, but my neighbor has, and he says they are big as cats. There's a load of rotten watermelons under my window and they smell like vinegar. But mostly things smell good: I stick my nose in my herb box every day. The basil and mint are heavenly. When I run my fingers through them I can smell it on my fingers. Yesterday I did some ironing and I put starch in some cotton shirts and skirts. The smell of the hot starch was so wonderful that I ironed everything in my closet—now all my clothes are stiff and crisp, but they smell fresh and clean too. I love the smell of laundromats in general now, and warm sheets and the smell of leather shoes in the back of my closet. I can hardly wait to get to the mountains and discover all the smells I've missed there the last two summers. Already I imagine how the cabins will smell, the dust and stone and old wood, old curtains and ashes, the horses and the grass and the flowers.

NEIL B.
The Doctor Said to Cut Back . . .

Neil B., with an M.B.A. in labor relations, is personnel director of a large corporation. His wife is an accounts payable supervisor at a bank. Both were heavy smokers, and they gave up smoking on the same day. Both are in their forties.

When we met, my wife had not smoked for five years. About nine months later, she picked up a cigarette again, and within a week she was up to a pack a day. We both smoked and smoked and smoked. I would say I was smoking two and a half packs of Marlboros a day.

The last year of my smoking, I got a sore throat on two or three occasions. It was only when I would swallow in certain ways, and it always went away. It would come for a while. Then it would go away.

The day I quit smoking, I went for a walk after lunch, and I coughed. It actually brought tears to my eyes, it hurt so bad. I did an about-face, went in and called my doctor, and asked him to recommend a throat specialist. That afternoon I took off from work and went to see the specialist. I remember on the way there, I thought, "Now he is going to tell me that I should quit smoking. And I am not going to do it." Every doctor says it: "You should quit smoking." And I got tired of that. I'd heard that so many times. They didn't understand my feeling. The thought of quitting caused me sheer panic. The thought of not having a pack of cigarettes in my front pocket just scared me to death. And the thought of never smoking another cigarette was something I couldn't even contemplate, it was so scary.

But when I was walking into his office, going into the examining room, I walked by a sign that said: "If you are contemplating quitting smoking, we have prescription drugs that can help you. Ask us about them." When I got into the examining room the doctor found a lesion on my vocal cord. He said he didn't think it was anything to worry about, it wasn't malignant, but it would probably help if I could cut back on smoking for a while. That was probably the best thing he could have said to me, rather than, "You've got to quit smoking!"

Something snapped inside of me at that moment. It was not fear. I didn't have a fear of this lesion on my vocal cord. But there was something that told me to quit. I said to him, "If you'll give me some drugs, I'll quit."

He said he would give me a prescription for nicotine gum. I didn't even know what it was that one took to quit smoking. My wife had been wanting to quit. She had talked about quitting, but I'd kept telling her, "No, no, I'm really not interested in quitting." So I said to the doctor, "If you give my wife a prescription, she'll probably quit too." Medicine being what it is, he couldn't do that. But he did give me a liberal prescription, and I could do with it as I chose, I guess. I assume this nicotine gum was not something dangerous.

I walked out of the doctor's office, got in my pickup and my cigarettes were on the seat beside me. I actually picked them up, but then I said to myself, "If you're going to quit, you had better not smoke this one." So I didn't.

On the way home I stopped at the drugstore, bought the gum, took it home, and set it on the table—I got home before my wife did that day—and didn't smoke. When she got home, I told her the throat specialist had found a lesion on my vocal cord and he was doing a biopsy to make sure it wasn't cancerous. He didn't think it was anything to be concerned about, but I had decided that I was no longer going to smoke.

I said, "I got you some gum, too." She said, "I'm not ready. This has happened too quickly. I'm not prepared to quit." I said, "I don't care whether you quit or not, I am. I'm done. And I'm never going to smoke another one."

That night, she smoked one more cigarette. I didn't even open up the gum until after we had had dinner. She had that one, last cigarette, and I chewed a piece of the nicotine gum.

When I wanted a cigarette there was a feeling in my chest that was only relieved by smoking. I assume nicotine caused that sensation. Well, when I chewed this gum, that feeling went away, and at that point I knew I had beaten it. For me, there were two parts to this habit. One was this feeling that I had in my chest, which was the need for nicotine. And the other part was, "What do I do with my hands?" I couldn't beat both of them at the same time. I had tried. I had tried quitting two or three times. Couldn't go a week. I was just climbing the walls. But I *could* handle one at a time, and that's what the nicotine gum made possible. It made the feeling in my chest go away.

Well, I chewed two more pieces that night. The next day I chewed the gum almost constantly. I had a burn from the tip of my tongue clear down into my stomach because of nicotine. The instructions said, "Chew it slowly," and I don't chew anything slowly, so I was tenacious even in chewing this gum! But it worked. It helped. I didn't have that physical need to smoke.

When I first quit I'd reach into my coat pocket for my cigarettes every time I reached for the telephone. It was such a habit, but I finally broke it. I was anxious to get rid of the gum because it struck me immediately that I had replaced cigarettes with this gum. I consciously started cutting back on it. My wife did the same thing.

Two months after we started on the gum, we were both taking some vacation time to work on a new house we'd bought. It's an hour and a half away from the city, where the prescription for the gum was. We were down to our last two pieces of gum. We had a decision to make: Were we going to take time out to go get gum? Or were we going to say, "The hell with it, that's it?" We talked about it and said, "That's it." So we quit the gum together, just the way we quit smoking together.

I started smoking when I was twelve or thirteen years old. I remember telling my mother how ridiculous it was that people became hooked on cigarettes and had to rely on these things. Shortly thereafter I became fascinated by cigarettes. I look back in old magazines, and in most of the photographs everybody's got a cigarette in their mouth. According to the ads, more doctors smoked Kents than any other brand when I was growing up. Older people, adults, smoked. There was quite a pressure to smoke, particularly if you wanted to grow up fast, and I did.

I had to put a lot of effort into learning to smoke, because in the beginning it made me sick. I began smoking Marlboros. I think that had as much to do with the Marlboro Man as it did anything else! By the time I graduated from high school, I had the habit.

Shortly after that I went into the Army. The Army at that time was particularly conducive to smoking. People who didn't smoke already started in the Army, because every break was a "smoke break." Army life was surrounded by cigarettes. There was no tax on cigarettes at the PX, so you could get them for practically nothing.

After I got out of the Army I went to college, and at that time cigarettes and coffee were very much in vogue at the student unions, the coffee shops. It seemed as though every university had three or four coffee shops, and the ones I went to were no exception. Adults smoked and adults drank coffee, and suddenly we were adults. You could tell we were adults because we smoked and drank coffee.

My first wife did not smoke. Throughout our marriage she disliked smoking and didn't understand what it's like to be hooked on them. I had absolutely no interest in quitting. In fact, I used to comment to people at that time that if a doctor told me that I had six months to live if I continued smoking, or forever if I quit, I would have been hard pressed to make a decision! That's how much I enjoyed smoking. At times my wife would tell me, "It would really be great if you quit smoking because it smells." I used to tell her that I smoked when we got married, and she was just going to have to accept that. I had no interest in changing.

The medical evidence—I'm amazed that one still hesitates to say "evidence"—but about five years ago I began to recognize that the evidence was overwhelmingly against smoking. At that time, too, the social acceptability of smoking changed considerably. Now it was:

You could smoke in a restaurant, and somebody might ask you not to. Being of the nature I am, I would probably tell them to go to hell. But at least I was becoming conscious that smoke probably did offend some people. The fact that smoking not only *didn't* turn me into the Marlboro Man—even after all those years of brand loyalty—but was, instead, making me offensive to people, began to bother me.

Finally I took a giant step forward and switched from Marlboros to a low tar: Merit. I had tried previously to go to various low-tar, low-nicotine–type cigarettes, but it didn't work. It didn't work at all. But I went to these Merits. After you get used to less hit . . . I don't know how to describe it, particularly for a non-smoker, but there is a feeling you get when you take a huge bunch of smoke into your lungs—there is a physical feeling when you do this. The lighter the cigarette, the lighter the hit. You have to get used to a lighter hit. Once I got used to that, those cigarettes were fine, but I smoked just as many, maybe more.

I certainly don't regret the decision to quit; I am very pleased that I quit. But I am pleased from a health point of view, which may have been what snapped inside of me. I suddenly said, "I've got to quit because of my health." I never had that kind of determination hit me before. Something swept over me that gave me that determination. Without it, I wouldn't have done it. Smoking has such a hold on you. You've got to have that determination. You've really got to believe you're going to do it.

Just no doubt in your mind that you can do it.

Since that time I have not even been tempted to smoke a cigarette. Now, that's not to say I haven't missed them. I missed a cigarette at lunch today. One thing that would make a non-smoker sick—as well as a smoker who still smoked—is that if today they decided that cigarettes weren't bad for you I would go down right now and get a pack of cigarettes, and I would start smoking probably two packs a day. I love to smoke. But I know I cannot smoke one, or I will smoke. So I am not even tempted to smoke. It is something like the alcoholic. One drink puts you back into it. There is no doubt in my mind that one cigarette would put me back into it.

I think one of the significant things is I never remember what day it was. People who quit a lot of times will say, "I have quit now for one year, two months, one week, and three hours," or something like that. But I still don't remember what day it was because that wasn't as significant to me as I was never going to smoke again. It has been over three years now.

Every night when I would go to bed I would cough a real deep cough, once, and then I would go to sleep. This was every single night. Also, if I would sing—you know how your vocal cords, when your volume is up, have a vibration to them? That would cause me to cough. And that's gone away.

Things that have not changed are the things that I was told would change. That things would taste better: I don't notice that at all. I would have more lung capacity:

I haven't noticed that. In fact, I had a doctor tell me, on a lung X-ray taken while I still smoked heavily, that he was amazed that I smoked, because my lungs didn't look as though I did.

The down side of quitting is that I have now, for the first time in my life, a weight problem. I *look* at French fries and I gain weight. Although now that I am understanding nutrition more, that might be a blessing in and of itself. French fries don't rank very high on the good nutrition list, what with all the fat and salt.

My wife is really bothered by being around smokers. She's an accounts payable supervisor. She has asked the people who work for her who smoke not to smoke in her office. The smoke really bothers her, where it doesn't seem to bother me.

I have not become one of those offensive ex-smokers. In fact, I eat lunch quite often in the smoking section. It doesn't bother me. If people want to smoke in my office, I don't care. People who smoke around me don't bother me. Now, at times though, the smell of smoke does, but I don't say anything. I guess my feeling is that if secondhand smoke is that bad for you, living in a city is just as bad, so I don't get enough secondhand smoke to worry about.

LISA M.
I Let Myself Smoke in My Dreams

Lisa, thirty and single, grew up on Long Island, New York, and now lives on the West Coast, where she works as a sales coordinator for a video game manufacturer.

I come from a family of smokers. As long as I can remember both my parents smoked heavily, and so did my aunts, uncles, and cousins. In fact, I don't know how my brother escaped. He is the one person in my family who doesn't smoke, and he absolutely hates to be around people who are smoking.

When I was twelve, I wanted to be cool, so I learned to smoke, to swear, and to do all those things that kids do to be cool. In college I smoked probably a pack a day, but by the time I quit—depending on how late I stayed up at night—I was smoking between a pack and a half and two packs a day. If I was at a party or at a bar drinking and up until two o'clock in the morning, then I would smoke about two packs a day.

I smoked for about eighteen years. I thought about quitting many times and I thought, "Well, when I really want to quit I'll quit." There were all kinds of reasons why I didn't want to quit just then. When I did try to quit, it was very half-hearted. I never really made that commitment, that decision to quit. I would quit for a couple of days or I'd have a cigarette here, a cigarette there.

Last Christmas I went home to New York. My great aunt—I was very attached to her—had just died of emphysema and she was a heavy smoker who refused to quit. She was seventy-five when she died, but for years she suffered and would sit in a chair and huff and puff but she would still keep smoking. And I could never say, *"Why don't you quit?"* because I still smoked.

My dad, who's fifty-eight, is a very heavy smoker too. In spite of the fact that he had a triple bypass a few years ago, in spite of the fact that he has high cholesterol, and in spite of the fact that he is overweight, he is still chain-smoking two packs a day.

While I was home for Christmas, my dad, my mom, and I were on our way out to brunch and my dad was smoking a cigarette while driving the car. He started to cough, that smoker's kind of cough, and got so red in the face he was purple. He couldn't get any air; but as soon as he could get his breath, he finished smoking that cigarette. *"That's it,"* I thought! So I rolled down the window of the car and threw my pack of cigarettes out. My dad said, *"What are you doing?"* and I said, *"I don't want to end up like you when I'm fifty-eight!"* I have not had a cigarette since.

It was frightening to me to see how my father was, and to realize that if I didn't quit I was going to end up just like that, as I know I am very much like him. Now I feel great, I feel I can breathe and smell the fresh air again!

The first week after I quit was easy because I was all fired up and that was it, *I was going to quit.* But after the first week it got a little bit harder, but every time I did feel the urge to smoke I would get this picture in my mind of my aunt, how she looked and how she could hardly breathe before she died and how she was so thin and so ill. Then I would get this mental picture of my father with that red face.

Those images would give me enough reasons why I shouldn't smoke. Then I'd give myself a mental image of my boyfriend and how happy he would be if I wasn't smoking because he cares and worries about me.

My uncle, who quit three years ago, said something to me: "Lisa, when you get a yen for a cigarette, and you really want one, that feeling is going to go away whether you smoke a cigarette or not, so why smoke a cigarette?" And I would think about that every time I got the urge for a cigarette and say to myself: "Okay, this is going to go away."

I still get yens for a cigarette but mostly when I am under a lot of stress. I'll be damned if after all this time I am going to start smoking again and have to go through the effort of quitting again at some later point in my life. This is it for me.

I dream about smoking all of the time. And I let myself smoke in my dreams. That is not going to hurt me. It is funny, because I know I am dreaming and I'm saying to myself: "If this wasn't a dream, I wouldn't be doing this." I know I'm smoking in my dream but that's okay: If that is where I gotta do it to keep off smoking, that's where I'll do it.

ANDY G.
A "Type A" Sort of Person

Andy G., now forty-nine, left an Eastern university to become director of athletics at a major university in California. His jurisdiction includes everything from football games to tennis matches, from physical education instruction to fund raising. It takes $19 million a year and a staff of over 150 people to get it all done. His success depends on the success of a lot of other people, especially athletes. Their attitude about smoking strongly affected him.

When I came to the West Coast I was smoking quite heavily. Smoking is stress related in my life: The harder things were, the more I wanted a cigarette, and the more cigarettes I smoked. Something happened to me when I smoked a cigarette that relieved, or that I thought relieved, my stress. I call it digital satisfaction. I smoked for about twenty years off and on, but when I smoked heavily, I chain-smoked. I was not only a heavy smoker but a heavy drinker as well. I am a risk taker, an entrepreneur, a type A sort of person. People like me operate aggressively; we're not afraid to take chances. We even take chances with our health and our lives.

About three or four years ago I realized I wasn't feeling very well. I was overweight and felt a great deal of personal dissatisfaction with almost everything. I chose to work on some things in my personal life. I quit smoking. I quit cold turkey; I just stopped. Two years later—I remember the exact day, in fact—I had my last drink of alcohol. Giving up these bad habits was an attempt to get some discipline and control in my life. I see smoking and drinking as related activities; I see them both as substance abuse. Nicotine and alcohol were substances I felt I needed, rather than something that I enjoyed.

I quit smoking because I didn't feel very well, and I thought that was unattractive. My wife's father died of lung cancer, and he had been a heavy smoker. My first boss in this business died of emphysema a few years ago, and he was a heavy smoker. I simply realized that it was stupid. I might die early anyway (I may already have smoked too much—I don't know how much damage I did, but so far my chest X-rays are good), but why *create* the reason?

I was also clearly influenced by things I had read, like the Surgeon General's report, the warnings on the cigarette packs, and the research that's reported in the newspapers and on television. It's hard to be ignorant of the dangers of smoking here at this university, with all the research on smoking that is being done here in our medical school, the committees that work on smoking policies in campus buildings, and stuff like that. People in California are very aggressive about not liking smoking. Those that don't like smoking *really* don't like it. They don't want you smoking around them, and they say so. I respect that. I don't like smoking around me now. It bothers me.

I can't think of a single athlete here at the university

that I have seen smoking. They are very aware that it would affect their physical performance. I know for a fact that a great many of them don't respect smokers and don't want people smoking around them. I'm sure their attitude influenced my decision to quit.

I remember the day I quit. I was in my office—I think I had burned a hole in a pair of pants, or knocked over an ashtray, or something—and I said to myself, "Stop. Just stop." I got up, walked out the back door, and threw the cigarettes (I think I had about seventeen cigarettes left in the pack) in a dumpster rather than throw them in the wastebasket in my office, because if I threw them in the wastebasket I could fish them out again. I threw them in a place where I couldn't get them back. That was it. I never smoked again.

I don't recall quitting as being traumatic; it wasn't something I needed to taper off or get counseling or help with. I just stopped. It was pretty easy for me the first few weeks because I had made up my mind that I wanted to give up smoking. Now instead of cigarettes I keep things around my desk that I play with, like Captain Queeg in *The Caine Mutiny*: I have a coin, I have a dish of rubber bands, and I'll just sit here talking with somebody, quietly twisting a rubber band.

I still get the urge to smoke—it comes and goes. I am nervous and intense during games. My job is very stressful because it involves the performance of other people. My success is dependent upon the success of lots of other people, and I find that nerve-racking. During the games, I have a straw or toothpicks or what-have-you, something in my hands that I can fool around with. That need hasn't gone away. I still need to cope with nervousness and stress, I am still a type A, I still take risks, but now I express those characteristics in different ways. That is what I mean by drinking and smoking being substance abuse. It wasn't for pleasure; it was a necessity.

It is incredible how much healthier I feel now that I have stopped smoking. After I stopped drinking, I felt even healthier. Looking back, I associated smoking and drinking. Now I attend a lot of Alcoholics Anonymous meetings. Talk about smoke-filled rooms! I was astounded at how many recovering alcoholics smoke. I am proud of the fact that I quit smoking and drinking.

MIKE B.
His Wife Had a Smart Idea

Mike B. is a successful businessman who was able to retire at fifty-five and to build himself an exceptionally well-equipped studio. He is a serious sculptor, calling on the influences of primitive art. He and his wife travel extensively to study ancient civilizations and primitive cultures.

It was such a trauma that I remember every detail of how I quit. My wife had been bugging me for seven years. She had smoked earlier in her life, and she had quit. One day she said to me, "I know you want a new Mercedes." We were going to drive our son back to college in Ohio.

"Instead of taking the old car, let's get a brand-new Mercedes, *but you can't ever smoke in it.* If you'll agree never to smoke in it, then I'll agree to buying the Mercedes." That was her way of manipulating me, and I agreed to go along with her.

My wife was very devious. She planned a three-week photographic safari through some of the most beautiful parts of Canada and the United States. She plotted a route up the California coast, across British Columbia, through the Canadian Rockies, down into Ohio to Oberlin, and then back to California through some of the great American national parks like the Grand Canyon. I went for it. If she hadn't used these incentives and said, "Let's get a new car," I think I would still be smoking.

Not smoking in the car was terrible. I went cold turkey after thirty years of three packs a day. I was very tense. I had never quit for more than half a day, and the trip took three and a half weeks. I kept my word: I never smoked a cigarette in that car. I screamed for three weeks, I was terribly irritable, but I never smoked cigarettes again.

The trip broke all my associative patterns, all my habits of going to work, smoking with coffee, smoking while making long business phone calls, smoking with drinking (we didn't drink on the trip since we were driving most of the time). We had a wonderful trip photographically, and I never once smoked a cigarette in that car. That car never smelled of tobacco.

We went up to Seattle and through Vancouver. I was cranky and kept getting worse, so I began to eat Life Savers. I consumed about five packs of Life Savers a day, maybe more. It gave me some oral gratification.

By the time we got to Ohio, I was much better; I was calming down. It took two weeks to get to Ohio, and the kid was being a pain, which is what teen-agers do for a living, and between him and me, my wife should be nominated for the Nobel Peace Prize. Anyway, we said goodbye to the kid in Ohio, and then my wife and I were together. It was a very nice time for us. I was a lot better by then, as we headed home. It took us a week. We went the southern route because it was already getting toward the middle of September. We stopped at a couple of the national parks, like the Grand Canyon.

The car was the device, the trigger, and it was a very clever one. We could have afforded the car anyway; that didn't have anything to do with it. It was just a gimmick. My wife is very clever. She knew that once I stopped, I probably would stay that way.

When I got home and was back in my office environment, I found it much easier than I had anticipated. I got a lot of reinforcement from people around me who had stopped smoking, although it was tough to have meetings with my staff if they smoked, but I learned to live with it. It was very hard to break the habit of smoking while I was on the phone. Two key associations I had with cigarettes were with coffee in the morning and when I talked on the telephone. These activities always prompted a cigarette response. Before quitting, I was on the phone all day, so I smoked all day. When I had a drink in the evening, I found that a very nice combination was vodka and a cigarette. That was a great combo and was very hard to give up. I have really missed it.

I dreamed about cigarette smoking for months. It still happens. I just had a dream last week that I was smoking, and I quit fourteen years ago.

I craved tobacco probably for three years after quitting. For a while, if people were smoking around me, I would say to them, "Blow the smoke at me, so I can smell it," because I loved tobacco. I ate two or three packages of mints a day for a few months, until my dentist told me to stop. I gained about five pounds.

I started to smoke in the Army. I was eighteen years old at the end of World War II, which would be 1944–1945. It was the fall of 1944, and they shut down all of the Army college programs and sent me off to basic training. In December of '44 I found myself in Arkansas with a gun in my hand, getting ready to go to the Battle of Bastogne to fill the battle lines.

Everybody was smoking, everybody. It was part of being grown up. It took me a couple of weeks before I was really hooked, and in the interim I got sick. It ruined my appetite and ruined my sense of taste.

Of course, I knew smoking could kill me. I didn't want to die of lung cancer or coronary disease. I have spent almost all of my life in the health industry, so I read all the medical literature. Before 1975 I had tried many times to quit. I quit twenty or thirty times. I tried everything. I tried gums and candies and everything. Nothing worked. I always went back to cigarettes. And I switched to mild cigarettes, but all I did then was smoke four packs a day instead of two. That is when Carltons came out, I think. I smoked Carltons, and they were terrible.

By 1975 I was ready to quit—I was forty-nine years old, I had been smoking thirty years, and my wife kept pestering me to quit. She made a nuisance of herself about how unpleasant it was, how bad I smelled, and how I was hurting my health. Then when the Surgeon General put all that stuff on the cigarette pack, it had quite an impact on me. I became convinced that there was a real problem here. I started to feel physiological changes. In 1970 a friend who smoked four packs of cigarettes a day dropped dead at forty-seven—that scared the hell out of me! I cut back for a while after that, but then I went right back to three packs a day.

I was a very nervous person in my work. I was always pushing very, very hard. I had a lot of feelings of inadequacy and anxiety about my work. In terms of position and responsibility, I was always way above what I felt I was trained to do. That was a pattern I always had. In those days I was vice-president of a major pharmaceutical company. It was a very nerve-racking job, because I was in an area that the rest of the company wasn't very interested in and I was trying to make it successful so I kept pushing, pushing, pushing—all of that created a lot of anxiety. I used cigarettes to help reduce the anxiety. The more anxiety I felt, the more cigarettes I smoked. They gave me a way to pause and think. There were a lot of wonderful aspects to that lousy habit.

In the seventies, after I left my position as vice-president of that pharmaceutical firm, I started a new corporation, which was very successful. Later, I helped a Chicago corporation go public, and that was a huge success; they make intravenous drugs for the hospital market. When I was fifty-five I achieved the financial target I had set for myself and I quit being a businessman to retire and take up sculpting seriously. I quit the boards of all my companies and I sold all my shares of stock.

The one real solid thing in my life was my good marriage. One thing that made me able to quit was the pressure from my wife and her support. My marriage was—and is—the most important thing in my life. For other people, it's their work or some hobby, but for me, it's my marriage.

In the fall of 1975 I quit smoking cigarettes. And I never had another. But ten years after quitting cigarettes, I started smoking cigars. I started in January of '85 and smoked for five months, until May. I was starting to do some excellent work in sculpture. I loved to sit and savor a cigar and sculpt. When I started smoking cigars, I thought I would smoke just one or two a day, but by May, I was up to twelve cigars a day so I quit again. I realized I could never touch tobacco in any form.

CELESTE HOLM
Smoking Was Chic

Celeste Holm's extraordinary acting career began when she created the role of Ado Annie in Oklahoma *and later replaced Gertrude Lawrence as Anna in* The King and I. *She won an Academy*

Award for Gentleman's Agreement, *and was knighted by King Olav of Norway in 1979—her title is Dame Celeste Holm. A public-spirited woman, she personally raised $20,000 for UNICEF (United Nations International Children's Emergency Fund) by selling her autographs for fifty cents—which means 40,000 autographs!*

I started smoking because in 1938 it was *chic.* I was four-teen years old, and I wanted to grow up. I thought smoking was a sign of growing up. It was absolutely idiotic, of course. I didn't know it could kill you. Nobody did. When I look back at it now, my Lord, I was fourteen! I see fourteen-year-olds now, with those eager little eyes, de-claring, "I'm grown up!" Well, they push it, and so did I. Some friends and I once decided to give ourselves a chal-lenge: to fill an entire shoebox with cigarette butts. It was ridiculous.

My friends and I didn't inhale when we smoked. The first time I ever inhaled was when someone gave me mar-ijuana. I was seventeen. I was at a party given by musi-cians, and somebody said, "Hey, I brought back some of those funny cigarettes from Mexico," and everybody said, "Whee!" They handed me one, and I did my usual number, and they said, "No, no, you're not doing it right. You've got to do *this*" [demonstrating inhaling]. It was astonishing. I immediately began hallucinating. I kept seeing clouds. I sat down on the floor, my back lean-ing against the wall, closed my eyes, and started seeing clouds in pink and blue rushing by at high speed. When I opened my eyes everybody was moving in slow motion. I passed the cigarette on to somebody else; one inhalation was enough.

I started looking for the guy who'd brought me to the party, and he was nowhere in sight. I found him in the bathroom in front of the mirror making faces at himself, like John Barrymore. At least, that's what *he* thought.

I said, "Take me away from here." He said, "Why did you bring me here?" I stared at him. I didn't know any of these people. I hated him. He hated me. Absolute paranoia, both of us.

We went into Walgreen's in the basement of the Times Building in New York. I went up to the pharmacist and said, "Somebody gave us some funny cigarettes, and I can't stand it, and I want to come back." The man behind the counter looked at me and said, "How old are you?" I said, "Seventeen." He gave us big bowls of chili and crackers and milk and we wolfed it all down. I still didn't like the guy I was with. But that's how I started inhaling. I don't think I ever would have inhaled if it hadn't been for that miserable experience.

I never tried marijuana again, but I smoked cigarettes for twenty years after that, inhaling every one. I never thought about it harming my health, or threatening my career, or even being offensive to anyone else. Many of my parts involved singing and dancing as well as acting, but I never considered what smoking might do to my voice or my wind. I don't know whether no one knew then what cigarettes do to your lungs and throat and larynx or whether it was simply that no one talked about it. In either case, I didn't draw any connection between the fact that I sang for a living and the fact that I smoked.

Twenty years later, in 1961, I was singing in Las Vegas. It was summertime, 104°F outside, 64°F inside, and I got what's called Las Vegas throat. It comes from going back and forth between the hot, dry desert air outdoors and the cool, moist, air-conditioned air indoors. The typical symptom is that you lose your voice. Speaking professionally, it means you have no middle register at all. The middle register is where you speak. I could sing high and I could sing low, but there was nothing in the middle. Here I was trying to make a living using my voice, and it wasn't there. I said, "This is dumb." So one day I stopped smoking, and I never did it again.

The first day I quit, I wanted a cigarette, but I said, "This is ridiculous." The second day I kind of wanted a cigarette, but I said, "This is silly." The third day I didn't want it that much, and the fourth day it was over. I stopped entirely. I never took another cigarette. I had no support group for this decision. What for? It was nobody's business but mine. It wasn't so much a health issue as a livelihood issue. I couldn't continue to earn my living as an actress and singer if I smoked. Once I realized that, there was no question in my mind. I had to quit.

I hate it when other people smoke. I'm offended by the smell. Smokers don't seem to realize that the smoke from their cigarette drifts around the room, so I just complain consistently. I move away from people who are smoking. They're affecting my life. I wish they'd go away. When people ask if I mind if they smoke, I say, "Yes."

ALLEN S.
You Can't Do It Until You're Ready

Allen S., forty-six, is president of a multinational corporation that manufactures and sells health products. Gradually he began to feel that it was an intolerable contradiction to be a smoker and part of a major health products manufacturer. He stopped smoking in 1984.

If I were like my wife, I'd still be smoking. She can smoke a cigarette or two a day or none; enjoy them if she has them, and if she doesn't have them, not miss them. She's never bought cigarettes, ever. When I stopped buying cigarettes, she stopped smoking. Where she is a very controlled person, I tend to be compulsive.

The first time I quit was about fifteen years ago, in the early seventies. I was about thirty, and I did it on my own, without getting involved in a group or cigarette substitutes or anything. I quit for one year, and I honestly thought I was over cigarettes and smoking. Then I began to believe that I could indulge myself with an occasional cigar after dinner. I often traveled for business, and I remember waking up in my hotel room and looking at the dresser across from my bed and seeing a large number of empty cigar five-pack boxes. I realized that I was smoking cigars the way I'd smoked cigarettes. I was going through twenty or thirty cigars a day, inhaling them, and using them exactly like cigarettes. I was smoking all the time, but instead of smoking cigarettes, I smoked cigars. It sort of sneaked up on me.

I had never made a conscious decision to start smoking again. I thought, "Well, I can have a cigar after dinner," and then, two cigars after dinner, and then all the usual habit triggers came into play—the phone ringing, or getting in the car. Eventually it came down to waking up in the morning and I'd have to have a cigar. When I saw all those cigar boxes in my hotel room, I said, "The heck with that. I'm going back to my cigarettes." Which I did.

The second time I stopped was in 1981 or 1982, while working for this corporation, before I became president. This is a company involved in manufacturing and selling healthful products, and I was under significant peer pressure to quit. I agreed to join a company-sponsored Smokenders program. I went to the meetings and I did all of the little things you're supposed to do each week to go through a controlled withdrawal. And I did stop smoking for a short period of time—about six months. I became such a miserable person—I was really unhappy. I made myself stop smoking by sheer force of will, but I never stopped wanting to smoke. It was awful. In fact, a group of people put up a petition in the Oakland office where I worked—I had several hundred people working for me—asking me to go back to smoking. Which I did.

There was no question in my mind that it was stupid to smoke. Here I was increasingly responsible for a company whose business is health and taking control of one's life, and I was embarrassed as much as anything. It seemed so completely out of character to be a part of this company, part of its management, and continue to smoke. It was a contradiction of everything the company stood for.

That I *should* quit had certainly been on the top of my mind for at least ten years before I actually did it. I had smoked since I was about thirteen. My father smoked cigarettes, and two of my four sisters did as well. My father quit, but by then I had been smoking for years. He quit long before I did. Most of my life—twenty-eight years of it—I was a steady, two-pack-a-day Marlboro smoker. The last few years I smoked Merits on the theory that they had less nicotine. The only result of switching to Merits was that I went from two packs a day to two and a half packs a day!

As my three daughters got older, the pressure at home to stop smoking became more significant, particularly since none of my kids smoked. They were very vocal about wanting me to quit!

When I quit this last time, more than anything else I felt I had come to the point where I'd had it. I didn't want to smoke any more, which was very different from all of the other times I quit smoking. Every other time I quit, it was because I felt I *should* quit smoking. I think I understand now why people say, "You can't do it until you're really ready." I don't know what you have to do to get really ready, but the biggest difference between the other times I quit and this time was that I *wanted* to quit.

One day about five years ago I told my family that I

would stop smoking when we left on our annual vacation—I always take the last two weeks of December off. I
told them in October that I would have my last cigarette
when that vacation started. I smoked right up through
the day we left. We were driving down to the desert from
San Francisco. As I got on to Highway 5, I still had a
couple of cigarettes left. I smoked down to the end of
that pack and said, "That's it, guys. I quit smoking." And
I did.

It was a good thing that I was going away for two weeks
of vacation. I was away from familiar surroundings, I was
away from the telephone, and I was away from the office.
That helped me get through the early part of it, because I
was in a no-pressure situation. I was away from all the
things that tended to trigger smoking.

I knew that I was never going to smoke again, and I
didn't. It was not that difficult. I never had the miserable
feelings or symptoms that I'd had at previous times.
What I did was gain thirty pounds, which I've had on and
off and on and off, but today I still have that same thirty
pounds on me. I gave up smoking for eating.

I've never had addictions other than food and cigarettes. I'm a compulsive person. I do things compulsively, and I know that. I work compulsively, I eat compulsively, and I used to smoke compulsively. I would
never fool around with anything like drugs that could be
addicting. It scares me, given that I know how compulsive I am.

One other thing happened that made me want to quit:
a friend of mine—a smoker—had a heart attack and

triple-bypass surgery. It happened less than a year before I quit. I remember going to see him at the hospital after he had his bypass. He had been a strong, robust guy, and he looked so weak and frail—and he was a smoker. I don't know if his heart attack had anything to do with the fact that he smoked—he may have had a lot of other things in his life-style or genetic background that caused it—but nonetheless, smoking was the thing he and I had in common.

When I went to see him in the hospital, it was awful. His wife was waiting in the hallway, wringing her hands. He was trying to put up a good front for his kids and me. He hadn't shaved in a while, he didn't have much strength, and he was lying there in a private room in a little hospital. I thought, "My God, this is awful." It was awful for him and it was awful for everybody around him. That really set my resolve to quit.

I always knew it was bad to smoke—you couldn't be a reasonably intelligent person and not know! I had seen the movies, I had seen the photographs, and I have known other people who have had heart attacks and cancer. You don't make it to my age in life without being exposed to that sort of thing, but seeing a close friend in that shape traumatized me in more ways than one.

I made several resolutions that day. The only one I've kept is the one to quit smoking. I also resolved to get back in shape and to quit working as hard. I still work very hard, and I am not in shape, but at least I don't smoke.

Now I hate cigarettes. I don't like being around smoke.

If I'm in a restaurant where someone is smoking, it makes me crazy. My eyes water. It is as though I have a strong, physical, allergic reaction to tobacco smoke. Still I must tell you honestly, I know if I had a cigarette I would be a three-pack-a-day smoker tomorrow. With all the knowledge, with all the resolve, with all the revulsion over cigarettes, I know for a fact that if I had a cigarette, I'd smoke again. I don't know what drug addiction feels like, but I think of the way that I react to cigarettes as an addiction. I know that as much as I hate them, that if I smoked even one, I'd be hooked again.

STEVE G.
Drinking and Smoking Went Together

Steve G. teaches English and history at a private boarding school, where he also coaches the soccer and basketball teams. His avocation is singing with a local opera company. A recovered alcoholic with fifteen years of sobriety, Steve is active in Alcoholics Anonymous. He quit smoking and drinking within a few years of each other. For a time he found A.A. meetings difficult because of "all the smoking."

In junior high school I was contemptuous of smoking and drinking, very puritanical, because I was an athlete. I was on all the all-star teams. But during the summer between the ninth and tenth grade I went through many changes. I lived in Los Angeles in a big house, and it seemed as though every room in the house had little containers of cigarettes. There were cigarettes everywhere, like candy in a candy dish; they were so accessible. My mother smoked, and my father smoked sporadically.

Anyway, I remember sitting there with a cigarette, playing with it and lighting it up a few times during that summer. It was something to do that was kind of taboo, since not many kids smoked during that period. There was no cancer scare. Adults said it would stunt your growth or cut down your wind, but I never experienced that.

I was a ninth-grader, at the top of the heap in a three-year junior high school. A three-year junior high allows you to make your mark, as you do in high school, unlike the two-year middle school system we have now. And then when high school started I was back at the bottom of the heap. Suddenly I wasn't the greatest athlete, there were 3,600 kids in the three-year high school to compete with, and the girls that I'd gone out with started going out with the senior boys. I felt rejected. On top of it all, I had to follow my older sister through the process, who was a saint—who *was* and still *is*—and who every teacher revered. I was constantly compared to her. I decided that I would be a rebel because I was not going to be cut from the same cloth as my sister. I started smoking when I entered high school; I was fifteen.

That sense of loss in going from the top of the pecking order to the bottom is why a lot of college freshmen start smoking. How many people never smoke until they are college freshmen? There's a tremendous vulnerability when you've been at the top and you have to start all over again from the bottom. Teaching school, I see it all the time, in seniors. High school seniors are often much more mature in their behavior than college freshmen are.

I continued to play sports and smoke clandestinely, because in those days if you got caught smoking you were off the team. But it didn't seem to affect my wind, so I continued to smoke. A lot of it was social. Everybody smoked Marlboro hard pack, because it was the macho thing to do. Although I think I was getting addicted, I didn't realize it at the time. I never even thought about quitting.

In the first year of college I became a serious smoker, and my drinking intensified. I couldn't imagine drinking without smoking—the two went hand in hand. About that time I began to have problems with alcohol. I was aware of it. I was getting in more and more trouble, but it was hard for me not to drink and smoke. At the end of my freshman year I was tossed out of UCLA for disciplinary reasons.

I went in the Army. Of course, smoking was a way of life in the Army. I smoked Camel non-filters, about a pack a day. It's funny, I never was what one would call a chain smoker. I would never light a cigarette and put it down and light another one. Smoking Camel non-filters, too: They were so strong, I didn't have to smoke that often. Again, it went hand in hand with the drinking.

I was stationed in France. Alcohol was readily available even though we were under age: It was very cheap. We would go to the EM Club every night after work, and we would smoke and drink. I smoked French cigarettes occasionally—they were incredibly strong. We could buy cigarettes in the PX for twelve cents a pack because they were tax-free. They were almost like fringe benefits. You could get a drink for five cents or ten cents during happy hour. If you were a compulsive-obsessive, as I am, it was a dream come true. You could get drunk on a dollar and smoke for practically nothing.

Anyway, smoking and drinking began to affect my health in my twenties. In the Army I began to have stomach problems. I also remember waking up coughing. Sometimes, with the combination of the alcohol, I remember waking up coughing and vomiting. I think one of the blessings in my life is that drugs—I consider nicotine a drug—affected me at an early age. I had very strong reactions.

My father died of cancer of the esophagus when I was about twenty-two. It was probably the most traumatic event of my life, and it accelerated my drinking. Three weeks after he died, I went to my first A.A. meeting, at the age of twenty-three, which was very young at that time. That was 1965. I continued to smoke, because in Alcoholics Anonymous the attitude was, "Well, you don't drink now, so smoking's okay." That was the prevailing attitude in Alcoholics Anonymous until very recently. You felt guilty if you didn't smoke at an A.A. meeting. After about six years of sobriety, by the way, I experimented with social drinking for a couple of years and it was disastrous. But I went to A.A. during that time.

I was smoking during that time, too.

I had quit drinking for a number of years, married, had children, graduated with honors, secured a teaching position, and felt comfortably successful, but smoking was still a very active part of my life. I taught in a boarding school. The majority of the people there did not smoke—the kids did, but the faculty did not. I taught English and drama and coached athletics. I probably smoked more at school than anyplace else. I would smoke when I rehearsed; I would smoke sometimes even in the classroom.

This was still prior to the real cancer scare and the real stop-smoking era. It was the late sixties, early seventies, when they were just beginning to make the connection between smoking and cancer. It was rumored that smoking stunted your growth. There were similar scare stories, too, that we whispered to each other when we were younger, something to do with masturbation stunting your growth as well. I always laughed at them. I often wondered how tall I would have been if I hadn't smoked or masturbated.

I still smoked probably a pack a day, but I started trying to quit smoking. I would go awhile without smoking, and then I'd start again. I was influenced by the fact that I was in a very healthy environment. Few adults at the school smoked; I lived out in the country; my wife did not smoke. It is marvelous that she managed to live with a smoker—I am now so intolerant of it myself. The smell, the ashtrays, and everything else.

My first major attempt at quitting was in my late twenties for six months. I ended up getting very heavy. Instead of exercising to compensate for the change in metabolism, I started smoking again. All it took was one drag on a cigarette and that was it, I was off to the races. In view of my experience in Alcoholics Anonymous, where you learn that one drink starts you drinking again, I should have realized that one cigarette would start me smoking again. And it did.

Probably the single most important event was Thanksgiving in 1972. We were invited to a party at this guy's house. He was a doctor. We went in, I lit up a cigarette, and he said, "I'm sorry, but you can't smoke in the house." Nobody had ever told me that before. It was a cold rainy day and everybody was inside; nobody else smoked. I went outside and smoked a cigarette, and I felt so alienated, so anti-social, so *excluded.* I had never been put in that position before. Nowadays it's quite common; lots of people won't let smokers smoke in their house or their office or their car.

This doctor was a cold bastard, very aloof, and I really hated his guts for making me do this. But years later, when I saw the same doctor, I told him how grateful I was because that was the turning point for me in terms of my attitude toward smoking. I had felt that alcohol was not socially acceptable—or more accurately, my *reaction* to alcohol was not socially acceptable—but I'd never felt that way about smoking. Cigarettes were always socially acceptable.

In February of 1973, for some unknown reason, I am not sure why, I just said, "Well, I am going to quit again." There was no preparation for it. I am sure this had weighed on my mind, but I was not aware of it. I did not set a date. I quit, and that was the last time I had a cigarette. I remember because I took a group of school kids on a week-long trip. It was the worst possible time to quit. I gave those poor kids holy hell. I was on edge; my nerves were raw.

I began to gain weight again, and this time I started running. I had gotten some exercise before, coaching the soccer and basketball teams, running up and down the sidelines. I decided to run every day, starting with a quarter of a mile. It was a good, healthy replacement habit. Although I gained weight, the exercise evened it out. I was in the best shape I've ever been in in my life.

I did some other things, too, which other people might find rather absurd. I would go to A.A. meetings and take carrots and celery to munch on. I ate junk food. That's a compulsion I have to this day, an addiction that I haven't quite got rid of, so my weight fluctuates.

And then I did something else. I realized that a lot of the pleasure of smoking was the oral gratification, the sucking. I had an infant at the time, so I took her baby bottle, put orange juice in it, and sucked on her baby bottle when I watched television in the evening. It worked! It had a tremendous pacifying effect.

I would never do this in public, but in my own house, when I'd come home after a hard day, it worked. The end of the day is usually the time I'm looking for some small reward. I couldn't drink. I could eat junk, but even that was hard because we lived out in the country. I'd take the baby's bottle, fill it up with orange juice, and I would sit there and watch TV, sucking on this bottle. It took a long time to drink orange juice this way because the pulp would clog the nipple. When the end of the nipple would get stuck with stuff, I'd clean it out and start over again. And it worked fairly well as oral gratification. I'm pleased to report that I did not become addicted to the baby bottle.

The key this time was not thinking in terms of quitting for the rest of my life; I quit one day at a time. I used the A.A. principles. I could smoke tomorrow without any problem. So rather than swearing off and making the "I'll never smoke again as long as I live" vow, I used the A.A. principles. That is what sustained me through the first year or two. Then, after two years, not smoking became a habit just as smoking had been.

It was very hard to go to A.A. meetings for a long time because of all the smoking. I would go home and I could smell the stale smoke on me. I would breathe it in. Sometimes I'd get headaches. I can see the danger of second-hand smoke. Fortunately, now there is a new consciousness in A.A., so there are lots of smoke-free meetings. I don't have to feel guilty.

My daughter now smokes! I notice teen-agers, particularly girls, smoke now. It's chic. When they quit they gain weight, so a lot of teen-age girls smoke to keep their weight down. It's become part of our cultural obsession with weight control.

My younger sister smoked. She's also in A.A., and she quit smoking and drinking. My mother quit a few years ago because of social pressure in her family. My mother had a tremendous weight gain after she quit smoking, which resulted in her having bad knees. Her knees couldn't support the extra weight. She's had some other health problems, too. It's been a mixed blessing. But she just couldn't stand the social pressure any more. The same with my mother-in-law, with whom I live. I think she quit because of social pressure from the family. It's nice to have her quit smoking because she smoked in the house.

People associate smoking and drinking; they have to do one with the other. A lot of people always have a cigarette with a drink. I come from a family of compulsive-obsessive people. There's a lot of alcoholism in my family and a long history of smoking. My father smoked, and he died of cancer of the esophagus. My mother and sister smoked until very recently. My uncles, my father's brothers, were alcoholic, and they all smoked. They all died of alcoholism.

I've had some wonderful benefits from quitting. I'm a singer. I sing opera. I'm a tenor, but my speaking voice has always been placed low. I also coach athletics after school, which involves a lot of yelling and cheering. I developed a tumor on my larynx, and I went in to have it removed. The first question the doctor asked me was, "Do you smoke or drink?" and fortunately I could say that I had been off both for a long time. He said: "There's no doubt in my mind that if you had smoked and drunk during that time you would have cancer of the throat now. Between the use and abuse of your speaking

176

voice from coaching and yelling without a megaphone or bullhorn, if you'd been smoking and drinking too, you'd have had cancer of the throat." It was one of those grateful moments where I could see that quitting made a difference. The tumor was nonmalignant, it was removed, and since then I have been singing and my voice is as strong as ever. That alone makes it worth it to quit.

BETSEY W.
A Compulsion Lasts about Two Minutes

Betsey W. took her degree in economics at a major university in preparation for the family business, from which she retired as president in 1987. Now she works part time doing public relations and assembling a history of the granite mining industry. She and her husband have been married since 1948. Gradually, she lessened the number of situations in which she smoked.

I always loved mountain hiking, so I decided that after I retired—in January of 1987—I was going to hike the John Muir Trail. It's over 200 miles of rugged mountain terrain in the Sierra Nevada in California. I knew I had to quit smoking in order to have the endurance I'd need.

I smoked my last cigarette the morning of December 31, 1986, and I told myself that I could have a cigarette again when I came down off Mount Whitney, the end of the John Muir Trail and the highest peak in the lower forty-eight states.

I'd smoked for about thirty years. I started when I was close to thirty years old, much older than most people. I had managed to resist smoking all through high school and college, though I tried my first cigarette when I was around fourteen. Four or five girls from my high school went to a friend's house. She had some old cigarettes, and we tried smoking them; they were pretty awful. They were all dried up. At any rate we tried them, and then we got worried that her mother would find out that we had been smoking so we put a lot of toothpaste in our mouths. Of course, we didn't have our own toothbrushes at her house!

But I didn't really smoke until much later. I was president of the family business in the early fifties and we were having a lot of conflict. My mother had been running the company and we asked her to leave. But she was suing us, and it was very difficult having her and her attorney at board meetings. Someone suggested that I smoke during these meetings because it gives you a chance to do something, to think for a minute, because the ritual of pulling a cigarette out of a package and putting a match to it gives you a little time. People will wait for that time, and you can get your thoughts together. So that's what I did. I smoked only at board meetings for a few years, then I started smoking more often.

I also had a housekeeper who smoked, and I admired her a lot. Smoking was something that I could do to be like her. A strange thing, but true.

I found it rather difficult to quit when I tried after a few years—so I must have been addicted. I eventually

smoked about a pack a day. I have always been a physically strong person—I have only been in the hospital
twice, when I had my two sons—and I thought I was the
healthiest smoker in the world!

Sometime in the early seventies I tried to quit smoking. I managed to stay off cigarettes from three to six
weeks. That sounds like a short time, but it is not a short
time for somebody who is quitting smoking. Once in a
while I would try—every New Year's I would think about
whether this was the year that I was going to quit smoking. Oh, but I didn't sign up for a course or any of that
stuff.

I don't think my husband has ever smoked a cigarette.
I don't think he even tried one when he was a teen-ager.
He didn't like to see me smoking. But I told him I wished
he would stop fussing with me about smoking. I think I
was smoking partly in defiance of his wanting me to quit
because I am a stubborn, defiant person. "I want to make
up my own mind, please!"

In November of 1985, I was thinking more and more
about quitting smoking. What I did first was to stop
smoking in places or situations where I was used to
smoking, and the first one was in the car. Now I admit
that I smoked before getting in the car and I would
smoke in parking garages when I got *out* of the car if I
drove up to San Francisco. I would always light a cigarette the minute I got out of the car, and that went on
through all 1986. I was still smoking, but never in the car.

Something else helped. Not many people at the company smoked any more. The few who did went outside

the building—their co-workers won't allow them to smoke in the office. My son had stopped smoking in September of 1986. When he told me that, it made me think even harder about quitting.

I disconnected myself from smoking at parties sometime during 1986. Cocktails and smoking were kind of a connection, but I managed to go to parties and not smoke. Some days I didn't smoke at work. I'd say, "Hmm, I went through the whole day without smoking."

The only thing I didn't manage to do in 1986 was to stop smoking when I got home, because my routine was to leave the office and stop by the grocery store every night on the way home. We eat lots of fresh vegetables, and when I shop every day at the same store I get to know the vegetables personally. I really do: I can recognize that they were there yesterday—they look the same, but a little older. Things like eggplant, a store has for days, and the eggplant waves and says, "I saw you before," and I say, "Well, you can stay here. It's nice seeing you again but. . . ." Anyway, when I got home I would put that bag of groceries down, pour myself a glass of wine, and light a cigarette. That is the only smoking I didn't manage to stop before the end of 1986.

I think there were times in 1986 when I got down to half a pack a day, but I was normally a pack-a-day smoker. I wanted to stop smoking and *had* stopped smoking in some situations on a trial basis. I was trying this and trying that in 1986. I knew I was going to retire at the end of 1986, and I wanted to do the John Muir Trail in 1987, but my breathing was not too good when it came to high altitudes. The John Muir Trail is over 200 miles long, all at high altitude!

I knew I had to stop smoking or I would never have the endurance to hike over 200 miles all the way to the top of Mount Whitney. In August of 1986 I had made some friends who were also interested in doing that hike. We started training together, and five of us went on a hike on the back side of the Sierras in August 1986. I had a terrible time. It's an easy hike, from Twin Lakes to Peter Lake, out of Bridgeport, northeast of Yosemite. Well, I didn't even get to Barney Lake, and that's only four or five miles from the trailhead. I began to feel terrible just before the switchbacks where the trail starts to get steep. I gave out before that, feeling awful.

I said, "I don't feel good. I don't think I should go any farther." The rest of them went up to Barney Lake, but I stayed and slept at the bottom of the switchbacks that night. I felt fine the next morning. I suppose it was the smoking and the altitude—about 7,000 feet—that made me feel the way I did the night before.

After that experience I knew that if I wanted to do the 211 miles of the John Muir Trail in one summer I had to stop smoking. One of the things that I hadn't done was the John Muir Trail. I decided that I was going to do the trail that following summer. I had to stop smoking, at least until after the hike. My son was going to meet me at Mount Whitney, and he was going to bring me cigarettes. That cigarette *after* the Mount Whitney climb was my dream.

I had figured that to do 211 miles it would take twenty-one days. But ten miles a day is a long way at a high altitude. You start adding some rest days, and it took us more time: It took us forty-one days. We had good weather. It didn't rain once. It snowed a little, and it hailed a little, but that's all. We washed everything we had when we laid over. We would dry some things, and then we would put on those clothes and wash the others. We'd start after each rest day with ourselves clean and our clothes clean, one way or the other.

We started the John Muir Trail on July 8, from Yosemite Valley. As we passed people on the trail they would ask, "How far are you going?" I'd say, "We're going to Whitney," and the fellow with us who had hiked a lot said, "Don't say that; you might not make it." And the three of us who hadn't done any of this before said, "Oh, of course we will. We won't make it if we *don't* say it. We have to keep that goal out for ourselves." It did seem impossible for the first few days. We reached the top of Whitney on August 17.

Before the trip I would say, "Well, you can't smoke today because you are going to do this hike next summer. You can't have a cigarette today." I knew myself well enough. If I had one I would smoke the whole pack. I mean, what are you going to do with the rest of them? I did say to myself, "I can quit smoking for seven and a half months until I get off Mount Whitney." Now I was up on Mount Whitney, and I never even thought about smoking one way or the other.

When we were coming down Whitney we met a lot of people who were going up, and we asked, "Can we get a cold beer down at the store when we come down off the mountain?" It isn't the beer so much as the coldness and the bubbles because that is different from the stream water. My husband met us at the end of the trail with a watermelon and lots of fresh fruit, and we went through that whole watermelon.

By this time, cigarettes were completely forgotten. Cigarettes were out. I had lost my interest in cigarettes as the hike went along, and I never did have that cigarette when I came down off Whitney. I haven't smoked yet, and I probably won't smoke ever again.

Oh, once in a while I think about smoking. My husband said something to me that was helpful: "You know, I have read somewhere that a compulsion lasts about two minutes." When I think about wanting a cigarette, or when I see a friend smoking, I sometimes think, "Hmm, maybe this cigarette will be what I hope for in cigarettes. Maybe I could ask her for a cigarette. . . ." Then my husband's suggestion runs through my mind. If I can live through one or two minutes, then the feeling goes away. I also pretend to smoke. Pretending smoking to me is deep breathing. So I take a few deep breaths, and I hold a pen as a cigarette and I play with the pen a lot. I wreck more pens because I pull them apart playing with them, and that is one of the things that I do instead of smoking.

Since I stopped smoking I have developed an addiction to corn chips. I used to smoke two or three cigarettes while I was cooking dinner and have a couple of glasses of wine. Now I have to have something with the wine so I eat corn chips. I eat an immense amount of corn chips. But I can get by without corn chips if there aren't any. It's not like cigarettes used to be where I'd have to go out and find some. Still, I do make sure that I have plenty of corn chips at home.

As a non-smoker, one of the things I notice now is that when I pass people in the grocery store I can smell if they're smokers. And it does not smell good to me. Now that I realize how bad people who smoke smell, I don't know how my husband, who never smoked, ever managed to stand me all those years, almost thirty years.

My next ambition is to do the Inca Trail in South America with a Stanford group. I was at Machu Picchu in the Peruvian Andes and I had such terrible altitude sickness—it's over 10,000 feet—that I never saw the ruins, even though I was very interested in them and in the sense of continuity of human beings going back hundreds of years in one place. So I want to go back again to see them.

I'm also going to do a shorter Sierra trip this year, 150 miles. It's twenty-one days, though, half the time of last year's trip.

One of the things I found out since I stopped smoking is that whatever I was looking for in cigarettes had never been there. I don't know how to define it exactly. It was the feeling of emptiness some people feel at times, as I did. But smoking never filled this internal emptiness. I kept hoping that the next cigarette would. But it never did.

JOHN G.
He Wrote Tobacco Advertising

John G. has been an advertising copywriter for almost forty years, on Madison Avenue and on the West Coast.

I quit smoking because it began to nauseate me that I was a slave to tobacco. My whole life revolved around being able to smoke. I even resented going to sleep because it meant I couldn't smoke. Concerts, the theater, movies, all were damned uncomfortable. I couldn't last longer than twenty or twenty-five minutes, thirty at the outside, before I had to run out to the men's room to have a cigarette. Of course, when I came back I'd have missed key parts of the movie. Say you have a ninety-minute show, and three interruptions of about ten minutes each, that's thirty minutes, or a third of the movie. I used to say the same thing to every person I ever went to a movie with. I'd say, "God, that movie didn't make much sense. It really didn't hang together." I didn't know who had died, and where the dog went, and why they were now in Alaska when they had been in Florida. . . .

And I hated the bookkeeping of smoking. When I took the dogs out for a walk, I had to tap my shirt pocket to make sure I had cigarettes, and then I had to check to make sure I had more than six cigarettes left. I had to check to see if I had my lighter, and be sure that I had matches with me in case my lighter didn't work. Maybe I'd better look to see if I've filled the lighter and have fresh flints. Heck, maybe I'd better take a fresh pack in case I get into a conversation with somebody.

My wife, now my former wife, was also a heavy smoker. We'd buy cigarettes by the carton, but still sometimes I'd have to go out at three o'clock in the morning, with a foot of snow on the ground, to some all-night diner that had a cigarette machine. Or we'd fish butts out of the wastebasket.

The amount of planning that smoking required was ridiculous. If I was going on a long drive, I'd have to remember to put an extra pack of cigarettes in the glove compartment. It was a constant preoccupation. It was crazy.

It wasn't even that I enjoyed smoking, but I was so damned uncomfortable when I *wasn't* smoking. If I had to go a whole hour without a cigarette I'd get a crawly, itchy feeling. It was terribly distracting. If I was at a lecture or in a meeting where I couldn't get out to have a cigarette, it wasn't long before I couldn't hear what the lecturer was saying. All I could think about was how much longer it would be until I could smoke.

I smelled like an ashtray most of the time, but so did almost everyone else. I started smoking when I was ten years old, sneaking off on Saturday mornings with my friends. We all knew we were going to smoke when we grew up; it was just a matter of when. My father was a physician and my mother was a registered nurse, and they both smoked. All the adults I knew did. There was much more acceptance for smoking then. It would never have occurred to anyone to ask you not to smoke or to tell you that they did not allow smoking in their house. It simply wasn't done.

It was considered bad form to light up during a meal between courses, but if I thought I could get away with it, I did. I always had a cigarette after meals. A cigarette, a cigar, a pipe, I used them all.

I always had a cigarette after lovemaking. That's a particularly agreeable time to have a cigarette. And with a cup of coffee; coffee and cigarettes just seemed to go together. The best cigarette of the day for me was the first one, as soon as I woke up. When you have a cigarette with nothing else in your system, it goes straight to home plate. It was nice. It felt good.

But that's remembering back a long time, because I haven't smoked for twenty-five years. I was a heavy smoker by the time I was sixteen, I smoked until I was thirty-two, quit for seven years, and then deliberately decided to start smoking again. I had put on some weight and I knew I was hitting the sweets pretty hard, and I remembered that smoking had cut my appetite. I thought if I started smoking again it would be easier to control my weight. I started out with two or three cigarettes a day, and within a week I was back to smoking three packs of Camels. I smoked heavily for a year, quit again, and haven't touched a cigarette or wanted one in twenty-five years.

I found a book by the late Herbert Brean, a writer for *Life* magazine, called *How to Stop Smoking*, which was very valuable. It's out of print now. I had tried to stop smoking several times and was unable to. I could make it maybe as much as two days without a cigarette by myself.

The book excited a different feeling about quitting in me; it changed my attitude. It's a funny book. The first chapter is why you *shouldn't* quit smoking. Then, if you read as far as the second chapter, he points out how essentially insane it is to allow your entire life to be dominated by a little white tube of paper with some chopped-up weeds in it. His key tip was that once you quit, pamper yourself in every other way you can think of so you don't feel sorry for yourself. For the first few weeks of quitting he says to take it easy on yourself with everything else— buy yourself some little thing you want, eat a whole bag of cashews, have a dessert with lunch. It's very wise advice because there is a terrible tendency to feel deprived, and if you do, you can't quit. Self-pity will wreck it every time. He made it clear that there are lots of things other than smoking that can make you feel good.

I realized what a grip tobacco had on me the first time I tried to quit. I hadn't had a cigarette for a week, and I went into a restaurant in New York for lunch. The service was typically slow and typically rude, really standard-issue stuff for New York, and I walked out in tears because I was sure they were being mean to me. God! I knew it must have been nicotine withdrawal, because even New York waiters had never reduced me to tears before. I was thirty-two years old.

Brean, in his book, was very cheerful and very optimistic. He said that you could quit if you sincerely wanted to, and he suggested telling everyone you knew that you were quitting. By telling everyone you created your own peer pressure to really quit, and you created a support system for your quitting as well.

He also suggested distracting yourself, so you don't sit around thinking about this great sacrifice that you've made. Go to four movies in a week, take up needlepoint, just don't think about what a poor, unloved child you are because you've quit smoking. And he tells you what a great sense of victory there is when you've finally quit. And it's true.

I've become a trifle fanatical about cigarette smoking, and especially about the calculated promotion thereof by people who ought to know better. The tobacco advertising I wrote in my days on Madison Avenue was tacitly, but clearly, aimed at the young. We knew that habit patterns in smoking tend to be well formed before one achieves maturity. It is a truism that rather few people start smoking after their mid-twenties. Today the ads depict people even younger than the models we used to use, and always with the theme that this is the passport to being "with it."

Promoting tobacco shows an unmistakable contempt for human life. No tobacco company could do well if its customers were moderate users. The five-cigarettes-a-day smoker is never the target market. The *heavy* smoker is the target, and we were never for an instant uncertain or confused about that when we were composing our lyrics.

We are so concerned about whales, sea otters, snail

darters, and the like that it seems just plain crazy for us to make so little protest in behalf of our own kind. If there were a movement to poison deer and peregrine falcons with toxins as potent and damaging as tobacco, a hue and cry would be raised that would jail the promoters of such a scheme overnight.

I don't write tobacco advertising any more; I haven't for many years, and I've become convinced that to do so is criminal. Quitting smoking is the smartest decision I've ever made.

STEVE W.
She Said, "Oh, You Smoke?"

Steve W. is president of a large business that has been family-owned for three generations. At the age of thirty-five, he shares the title of president with his brother. He has a master's degree in psychology and enjoys skiing as a sport. He never thought about quitting until he actually did quit.

I know a lot of smokers who have tried to quit a lot of times and to them "trying" means not buying a pack of cigarettes, and then not having any cigarettes for a whole morning or maybe a whole day. I always said to myself if I ever wanted to quit I would quit and never smoke again. I didn't know if I was fooling myself or not, because I had never tried.

I had a kind of a nagging, half-conscious concern about my health, but never really up front. Besides, it was always easy to find an older person, eighty or ninety, who was smoking, and with that I could justify all the cigarettes I'd ever had, and was going to have.

My mother was a smoker, too. She recently quit smoking, and I think that she is one of those people who have tried to quit, which means that she has set down cigarettes for weeks, even months, over the last ten years, and then has started smoking again.

When I finally quit I had smoked for about twenty years. I would say I probably had my first puff of a cigarette when I was fourteen. Some older kids had cigarettes that they had taken from their parents and would pass them around in a hideaway, dark-alley–type situation. It was exciting to sneak a puff of a cigarette.

I didn't really like it at first, because it burned my throat and made me cough, but I figured it was something to overcome, like other adult tastes. In the very beginning I probably smoked once or twice a month. Then there was a gradual increase up to about a pack and a half, maybe even two packs per day, when I was about seventeen. It took three years to progress—if you can call that progress! I smoked at that level until I quit two years ago. I quit because I'd gotten a date with a very pretty girl.

It happened that I asked this girl, Janet, to go out with me. She was very, very pretty, and I was very much attracted to her. She was quite health conscious—health club every day, health foods, but not overboard. I knew she would have nothing to do with me if I smoked, and so the night I was to take her out I brushed my teeth fifteen times, washed my hair six times, put on a clean set of clothes, and did not have a cigarette on the way to pick her up, did not have one the entire time I was with her that evening.

Janet didn't know I was a smoker. I had cleaned my car very well. She spent the night at my house that evening. We didn't have sex, but we did share my bed because we had had a lot of wine and she didn't want to drive home. It was a very clean first date—no sex. When we got up that Sunday morning, she made some breakfast and we sat out by my swimming pool in the sun, and we were just going to have a relaxing day around the pool. Meanwhile, I hadn't had a cigarette. I had never gone that long without a cigarette since I was around sixteen or seventeen, when I got to the pack-and-a-half deal. And I said to myself, "Well, I like her." It was then about two o'clock in the afternoon, and I still hadn't had a cigarette. I had a cup or two of coffee, and so the need for the other half of that experience—a cigarette—was very much there all morning.

Finally I said, "Oh, hell. Either she likes me for who I am, or she doesn't." I went into the house, got my pack of Camel filter cigarettes, went out by the pool, and said, "Oh, it's about time for a cigarette." And she said, "Oh, you smoke?" And I said, "Oh, occasionally." I didn't want her to know I was a big-time smoker. I lit it up and got about halfway through the cigarette, which is maybe four or five puffs, and I could literally feel the drug of the cigarette taking hold. I could feel my body getting very small shakes.

She didn't say anything, and I didn't say anything to her, except, "This cigarette isn't that great." She didn't know that it was unusual for me to put a cigarette out half-smoked, or to react to it like that.

Tuesday night of the following week, I went to dinner with her again. I still hadn't had a cigarette. I was still sticking to the commitment that I don't need to have that shaky feeling and I don't need all of the other negative things that go along with cigarettes. It wasn't a health decision—it was more cosmetic. Cigarettes make you smell like an old ashtray. They mean your teeth get brown—I have pretty nice teeth. Plus all of the other things that go along with smoking.

That pretty girl that first night was the inspiration. After our second date, she put a pack of candy cigarettes in my mailbox because I told her that, indeed, I was a more-than-occasional smoker. We were having fun with her bringing me candy cigarettes.

The first three weeks of not smoking I was concerned that I wouldn't be able to go through with it, because some of the people in my office who noticed I wasn't smoking—there was no cloud of smoke billowing out of my office door—began to make me think that there were going to be withdrawal symptoms. My secretary was saying, "Boy, you're irritable," and I thought, "Well, hell."

Some of my friends who had paid a lot of money for Smokenders' seminars brought me stacks and stacks of literature about what types of withdrawal symptoms to expect. Irritability is one of the things to watch out for, and some of my co-workers told me that I was a grouch. Either I was having a physical withdrawal to not having a cigarette or it was purely psychological, but at any rate, within two months I was more or less back to my old self.

After reading all the literature on smoking and hearing about everyone else's problems with quitting, I thought, "My God, maybe I do need some props." I went out and bought a whole bunch of Life Savers and gum, and I found myself eating more. I don't know if I really needed to or if it was because of the influence of all the damn literature. I quit and then I started reading the literature and thought, "Well, hell, I had better have some Life Savers in my pocket." Sometimes I feel that I would have been better off without reading all that literature!

I never broke down since that half a cigarette the first day, although I have smoked two cigars without inhaling since then. That was on a weekend in Las Vegas. With lots of cocktails, it seemed like the time to have a very expensive cigar, and I smoked two of them, one each night. That was about a year after I'd quit. I have not smoked since, and I mean no cigars either!

I know that now I have a lot more lung capacity. Skiing is one of my greatest physical exertions every year, and now I can go down hills where I used to have to stop three or four times to catch my breath. I think it is just great—my excitement in skiing is not held back now. I can do more, and that is great.

In the last year and a half I have had three or four dreams about smoking. I have waked up and said to myself, "Crap, I've had a cigarette; in fact, I've had several." And then I tell myself, "Oh, hell, it was just a dream." But still, I feel really bummed out that I let a small urge to smoke overcome my greater need not to.

An interesting point: Most of the people I know try to quit smoking by eliminating the accessibility of cigarettes. They don't have a pack of cigarettes in their desk drawer, in their car, in their shirt pocket. I have given this kind of quitter many a cigarette! I think that's ridiculous. When I went out with that girl, Janet, the first night, I had a full pack of Camel filters, my favorite brand at the time, in my car. I had that full pack in my kitchen that night, and of course, the next day, that Sunday afternoon, I had a full pack of Camel filters. That same full pack was in my shirt pocket for the next six weeks. I never had that cigarette pack out of my reach. It dwindled because my friends who were continually in and out of my office would bum cigarettes from me. Eventually, the pack was finished, but not by me. It was a nice, secure feeling that if I ever had one of those situations where I *had* to have a cigarette—I could light one up. But when my friends finally bummed all the cigarettes in that pack, I never bought another pack.

My daily routines, such as checking to make sure I had a pen in my top pocket, my wallet in my back pocket, and my comb in my right back pocket, used to include making sure that I had a pack of cigarettes and a pack of matches. Now I've eliminated two items in my life, which is a great freedom. When I "pack up" in the morning, I don't have to look around for cigarettes and matches.

Other habits have changed, too. I drink a lot less coffee now, probably 30 percent of what I drank before. Over the last ten years that I smoked, I was probably drinking eight cups a day—and I am talking mugs, not tea cups. Now, two or three at the most. Interestingly enough, I now get mild headaches from coffee if I drink "too much," which I didn't when I smoked.

Now, after I get home from a nightclub, or a bar with a band for dancing, and I smell my clothes, I think, "My God, I was wearing these? They smell so horrendous from the cigarette smoke."

Why did I quit? My quitting was kind of an accumulation of disliking my clothes and my hands smelling like cigarettes, combined with the probable health consequences of smoking—death. It all just came to a head on that date. People used to tell me that if I didn't smoke I wouldn't be limited as to the type of girl that I could go out with. Well, I found out that was total bullshit because now *I* will not go out with smokers. I'll only go out with girls who don't smoke.

CHRIS S.
For a While I Quit Quitting

Chris S., twenty, is assistant manager at a gourmet coffee and tea shop. He is a college student majoring in business administration. He found out that smoking is less attractive for people in his age group than it used to be.

I knew smoking wasn't very good for me. I knew people died from smoking cigarettes. I just figured I would quit when I wanted to. I would do it for a few years and quit. My father had been telling me for years to quit smoking, but I didn't listen to him. I said I would quit when I was ready. I knew I could quit sometime, but I got pretty nervous for a while when I was smoking two packs a day and found out that it was going to be harder to quit than I thought.

I had tried smoking when I was in third grade with my cousin, trying to be cool, but I hated cigarettes. My parents smoked. My dad quit, but when my parents got divorced he began to smoke again. I lived with my father and stepmother. My father finally quit again about two years before I started high school. I was the one who got him to quit. I kept telling him how bad smoking was and everything.

When I started high school the crowd of people I hung around with all smoked, so I started smoking. That was

197

in Ohio. When I moved to California to go to high school here, I smoked more than ever. I smoked Marlboro Reds. I started to smoke at fourteen and stopped just after I turned twenty—that's about six years of smoking. At the end I was smoking about a pack a day, but when I was working at a gas station, where all I did was sit in a box by myself, I smoked almost two packs of cigarettes a day. Everyone at the gas station smoked cigarettes. I went back to one pack a day when I began to work in this coffee and tea shop.

I had quit before and started again, and quit and started, and then I pretty much quit quitting. It hadn't worked out. I switched cigarettes, went to light cigarettes, smoked only a few a day, and then I just went back to my normal Marlboro Reds, smoking a pack a day. I figured I would quit when I wanted to quit.

And then one day, out of the blue, I decided that when I'd finished the pack I was smoking I wasn't going to have any more. I had one cigarette left though, just in case I needed it, but I've never had another one since then. I kept that one cigarette around for about two weeks and then it disappeared. Someone took it from my room and smoked it or something.

I feel a lot better since I quit. For the first few weeks I almost seemed sicker, I coughed more, but I guess that was my body just getting over it. I think I am still recovering from the years of smoking, but in the next few years I should be a lot healthier.

It was tough at first, but I didn't have many withdrawal symptoms. Wanting to have a cigarette was on my mind constantly. Some of my friends still smoked, and it was hard when I saw them smoking. But gradually I just got over it. Then three or four of my friends quit smoking too. They all quit after me, and none of us have smoked since. We are all about the same age, but I believe they had smoked for a shorter time than I had. They were about a year and a half younger than me, so they hadn't smoked quite as long or quite as much.

I quit on my own. I didn't have any withdrawal that I can think of, except that mentally I wanted to smoke. But I kept saying, "I have gone a day, so I will go another day; I have gone two days, so I will go another day." Now I have gone four or five months, and I don't even think about smoking. I actually view smokers as sort of outcasts. They seem different from everyone else. I see someone smoking, and it just doesn't seem natural or right, whereas before, a cigarette was like part of my body. I had one going all the time. Now I don't like people smoking in my apartment. If people are going to smoke, they have to go outside.

Smoking now seems to be more of a teen-ager–type thing. It is getting less and less popular in my age group—twenty, twenty-one years old—but I still see a lot of high school kids out in front of schools sneaking a smoke.

ELTON W.
He Changed His Attitude about Quitting

Elton W., a magazine editor for many years, is now director of public relations for an advertising firm. In his late forties, he also is a dedicated fly fisherman and photographer, having won numerous awards for his photographs.

I tried to stop smoking any number of times before I finally quit. I would make little deals with myself: "Today I am going to not smoke." That would last until about eleven o'clock in the morning. Or I'd decide I'd only have a cigarette if someone offered me one. In those days, the correct cigarette protocol, if you were going to smoke, was to offer anyone in the immediate vicinity a cigarette, too. Sometimes I'd deliberately not buy cigarettes and just mooch instead. That never lasted very long. Eventually some exasperated colleague would say, "Why don't you buy your own damn cigarettes?" I switched brands. I tried filters. I tried low-tar cigarettes. Those had an interesting effect: I went from one pack a day to three. Just as much tar and nicotine and three times the oral gratification. I tried quitting when I was out of town on assignment in remote locations. All I accomplished was feeling wretched, sleeping badly, and coming back thoroughly miserable. I tried smoking a pipe and once, very briefly, cigars.

I was the classic quitter. I knew everything there was to know about quitting. After all, look at how many times I'd done it. I tried every trick in the book. It's a good thing I never had access to classified information. All they would have had to do to get me to tell them every-thing would have been to take my cigarettes away. "Here are the atom secrets, just give me a cigarette." I wanted to quit for several years before I actually started trying to quit, and I tried to quit for a couple of years before I accomplished it.

And yet in thirteen years of smoking I never bought more than two packs of cigarettes at a time. A carton was more of a commitment to smoking, more of an admis-sion that I was addicted, than I was willing to make.

I used to say that I belonged to the caffeine-nicotine school of writing. My cup of coffee was on the left, my cigarettes and ashtray on the right, and my typewriter in the middle. When I would try to quit I'd go through all the symptoms of withdrawal—anxiety, irritability, insom-nia, hyperactivity, an inability to concentrate—to the point where I couldn't write. I was secretly terrified that I couldn't write without cigarettes. That was very scary since that's how I earned my living!

The discomfiture was extreme for weeks. On a number of occasions the withdrawal symptoms were so disabling that I started smoking again just to be able to function effectively. It wasn't weakness of will; it was simple prac-ticality. I had a family, and I had to be able to earn a living. The discomfiture does fade, but it fades gradually over a period of five to six weeks. It was a couple of months before I felt good about my writing again.

There's a certain amount of evidence that I did not handle my various attempts at quitting with all the charm and savoir-faire with which I ordinarily conduct myself. On one occasion, when I was five days into quitting, my wife went out and bought me a carton of cigarettes. She presented them to me with the announcement that she didn't like my smoking but she'd rather I smoked than continue to behave the way I had for the past few days.

I started smoking when I was thirteen or fourteen because my best friend had started. The crowd we traveled with was bright and precocious, and smoking was one of those sophisticated affectations that made us feel independent and adult. We were in our sophomore year of high school.

Smoking was a difficult habit for me to acquire. It tasted bad, it made me cough, and it burned my throat. That was a bit of an obstacle to overcome, but I persevered in the name of social *panache*, and within a few weeks I was walking around with a pack of cigarettes in my pocket all the time.

Cigarettes were ubiquitous when I was young. In the world I grew up in, the majority of adults smoked, though my father didn't, and my mother smoked only socially. All the actors and actresses in the movies smoked and they looked sophisticated, so I was sure that eventually I would, too. Judging from what we saw on the screen, practically every social situation was enhanced by a cigarette.

I practiced appropriate facial expressions and ways of holding the cigarette to appear properly jaded and elegant. My mother told me plainly I looked foolish, and she was right. My father, a doctor, told me smoking wasn't good for me—cigarettes had been called coffin nails for many years before I started smoking. He also told me I'd probably outgrow it, which, given the fact that I wanted to appear adult and not as though I were going through another adolescent phase, was an excellent strategy.

By the time I graduated from high school, I had the habit. I was smoking a pack or pack and a half a day, and I smoked all through college. I went into journalism, working at one of the largest magazines published in the West. I don't know that the journalism profession is inherently high-stress, but my reaction to it was high-stress. I was very driven, and I worked very hard.

Still, smoking did serve some useful purposes in the thirteen years that I smoked. It gave me something to do with my hands. Now I fiddle with pens or shred Styrofoam coffee cups or play with my glasses. It also allowed me to look thoughtful. When someone would throw me a question for which I didn't have an instant answer, I would take out my pack of cigarettes, carefully select one, tap it to pack the tobacco, fumble around for matches or my lighter, light the cigarette, inhale deeply, and by that time I'd have thought of something to say. And I looked as though I was considering the best approach instead of scrambling madly for a response. Pipes are the best for that purpose. A good pipe smoker can

stretch out the ritual for two or three minutes with practice. Properly managed, a pipe can increase perceived
I.Q. by twenty-five points.

What finally made me determined to quit was editing a
college text called *The Psychophysiology of Respiration and
Lung Disease* for a friend. The chapter on emphysema
opened with the lines, "No one likes an emphysema patient. Their doctors don't like them, their families don't
like them, and they don't like themselves. Their doctors
don't like them because they don't get better. Their
families don't like them because strong emotion can trigger an emphysema attack, so emphysema patients typically become cold and withdrawn in an attempt to fore-
stall an attack. And they don't like themselves because
they don't dare express their strongest feelings." That
sounded like a rotten way to spend the last years of life. I
smoked steadily the whole time I was editing the book,
and when I was done I smoked one last cigarette, and
that was it. I had been smoking a pack or pack and a half a
day for thirteen years.

At the time, two things conspired to make me successful. I had received a promotion, so I was in the process of
winding up my old position without having yet taken on
any major projects for my new one. There were no criti-
cal deadlines for a couple of weeks.

The key thing was that I changed my attitude toward
quitting entirely. In all the previous attempts I acted out
of a spirit of self-sacrifice. I was giving up something that
I liked and quitting was unpleasant. I felt like a real martyr. I'd go three days without cigarettes and feel as

though I deserved the Congressional Medal of Honor *and* the Nobel Peace Prize.

This time I didn't. I had to commute across the bridge every morning, so as soon as I hit the bridge I started saying out loud, to myself, "No, thanks, I don't smoke." I'd imagine myself in all kinds of situations where people might offer me a cigarette, and then I'd say, out loud, "No, thanks, I don't smoke." Not, "I'm trying to quit," but, "No, I don't smoke." I was practicing, trying on, inventing a new identity for myself, as a non-smoker. Not an "ex-smoker" or a "reformed smoker" but a *non-smoker*. I imagined this super-wholesome, super–Boy Scout persona for myself, the sort of person who would *never* smoke. I was a Boy Scout leader at the time, so I pretended that I was the kind of squeaky clean purist who would be shocked and offended by smoking, the sort that people would hardly even think of offering a cigarette to. I imagined this person as a real Goody Two-Shoes, but I don't think I ever took it that far in reality. That was just for the person I was creating in the car on the commute twice a day: "No, thanks, I don't smoke." God knows what the other commuters thought of me smiling and nodding pleasantly and obviously talking to myself every morning and evening.

I also kept a generous supply of carrot sticks and celery sticks around to deal with the oral gratification issue. In the past I'd tried chewing gum, but since I hate chewing gum it didn't work very well.

I haven't smoked in over twenty years. It's not a struggle at all. In fact, I find that now that I no longer smoke

I'm offended by the smell of tobacco on someone's clothes or hands or hair. I've even checked out of hotel rooms rather than stay in one that smelled of tobacco. I guess I just outgrew it, exactly as my father said I would.

ARLENE H.
I Had Lost Control of My Life

On Arlene's twenty-third wedding anniversary, her husband announced that the marriage was over and walked out. The next day a postcard came in the mail from the local hospital announcing an introductory open house for people who were interested in quitting smoking. Arlene had smoked for thirty-two years, but, as she says, "I didn't have any plans for that evening. I didn't have any plans for the rest of my life. So I went."

It was like beating cancer. It was like climbing Mount Everest. It was one of the most incredible experiences of my life. Everyone who knew me well said, "Arlene, I can't believe you did that!" And that made it even better. The last cigarette I had was January 14, 1985. I have never had another puff on a cigarette. I have no desire to smoke. Occasionally, a particular place or particular people will trigger a memory of when it was comfortable for me to smoke, but I don't want to go through all the rigmarole of smoking again. It isn't worth it. I'm more comfortable *not* smoking than I ever was smoking. To this day, my daughter celebrates that anniversary. She sends me a card and takes me to lunch. She's very proud of the fact that I quit.

I started smoking when I was fifteen and a half. My parents had said that I could not smoke until I was sixteen, so the day I turned sixteen, I walked into the house smoking a cigarette. My parents couldn't figure out how I'd learned to smoke so fast. Well, I'd been practicing for six months, that's how.

I wanted to smoke because all my friends smoked. We thought it was really neat. It was adult, sophisticated. The older kids smoked, and we wanted to smoke, too. The athletes smoked. Everybody smoked. But for all my desire to be sophisticated, it was very difficult for me to learn to smoke. I coughed. I got sick. I almost threw up. It was very difficult to inhale. It was awful. Now I realize that I was introducing a foreign substance into my body, and my body didn't like it. It never occurred to me that it was bad for me.

We smoked all the time as kids. When we were studying, walking to school, in the car going to football games, at the movies, everywhere. As I got older, I smoked more. At work, my pack of cigarettes was right there next to my typewriter. I smoked going to work, we always went out for a drink after work and I smoked there, I smoked going home, wherever I was, I smoked. I was smoking a pack and a half a day when I quit—and I'd been smoking for thirty-two years.

I would never leave the house without being sure that I had at least two full packs of cigarettes, just to be sure I didn't run out. I always carried an extra pack or two of cigarettes. I bought cigarettes by the carton. If it was eight o'clock at night and I had only one pack left, I'd go to the store and buy a new carton. It was too frightening to run out of cigarettes. I think I only ran out once, when someone came over and they were smoking my cigarettes. I was being polite, but I kept thinking, "What if we finish this pack? What am I going to do?" I was really angry.

Now lots of stores are open twenty-four hours, but I had been known to drive quite a distance to find a store that was open before that was true. Mostly it was to be sure I'd have cigarettes for the next day, just in case the forty-day flood came or some other calamity occurred. It was so time-consuming to be constantly planning, pre-planning, to have enough cigarettes. I also had cigarettes in three or four different rooms of the house. I had a pack in the bathroom, a pack in the kitchen, a pack in the living room.

Now that I am able to be honest about it, I don't think I ever really enjoyed smoking. I enjoyed the situations in which I smoked, but smoking did not enhance them or make them any better.

I smoked from the moment I got out of bed. I couldn't talk on the phone without a cigarette. I couldn't write a letter without a cigarette. I smoked when I was angry. I smoked when I was happy. Sometimes when I couldn't smoke for one reason or another I'd long for one, but when it was over I'd think, "I feel so good not smoking. What if I didn't smoke?" But then another voice would say, "Aw, c'mon. You deserve it. Be good to yourself," and I'd light up. I think truly the more you smoke, the more you want it.

Other times I'd wake up hating the taste of tobacco in my mouth. I remember not feeling good in the morning. I'd worry about my coughing. I'd think, "It smells so bad, maybe it would be great if I didn't smoke." I'd make myself little promises, like, "Today I'm not going to smoke until five o'clock." Within twenty minutes I'd have a cigarette in my hand. And then, of course, I'd beat myself up for being so weak. I thought about quitting for ten years before I did it.

My family wanted me to quit, too. Neither of my children smoke, and my ex-husband quit a three-pack-a-day habit cold turkey fifteen years before I quit. I tried quitting with him. He smoked cigars, I smoked cigarillos, but then I went back to cigarettes. They all wanted me to quit. My daughter was dating two boys in med school and they would talk to me about it. I kept saying, "Look, I smoke and it doesn't affect me. I don't think you understand. I walk and I run and I play tennis, and smoking doesn't affect me." I was convinced that smoking did not affect me because I was a very strong person and my lungs were extremely strong. My final rationale was that I could be run over by a truck tomorrow, so what difference did it make?

Then my husband announced on our anniversary that our marriage of twenty-three years was over, and the next day I got this little postcard about a behavior modification course to quit smoking. They were having an open house to talk about their method for quitting. I thought, "Well, I don't have anything to do for the rest of my life. I have no plans. I might as well go." I was *so* depressed.

I went down to this portable classroom in the hospital parking lot, and there were 120 people there, all coughing and smoking. It was a wary group. We were all just going to look. The people offering the course never talked about quitting. They talked about smoking and why we smoked, and everyone laughed a lot—and smoked. They talked about getting a flat tire, so you have a cigarette, but when you're done with the cigarette, the tire's still flat. That really hit home. Everyone groaned with recognition.

I signed up. I was willing to give it a shot. It was the only positive thing I could think of that I could do for myself. I had totally lost control of my life. My husband was gone. My children were gone. I was alone for the first time in twenty-three years. I was a lost soul. My friends all thought I was insane to try quitting when I was under so much stress. They thought I should smoke *more,* have another drink, kill this pain. I thought maybe they were right, so the first night I went up to the instructors, poured out the whole story, and asked if they thought this was a good time to try quitting. They said it was a perfect time, because the whole point of the behavior modification is to get you to change your routine. There is no better way to change your routine than to discover quite unexpectedly that you are no longer married after twenty-three years.

It *was* perfect. It distracted me from all the pain because I had to concentrate on not smoking. We had homework assignments every day, like calculating how much we had spent on cigarettes—mine came to *$15,000!*—and how much we were likely to spend over the next five years, ten years, fifteen years. We wrote down when we smoked every single cigarette, and why, for a week. We got buttons that said, "I choose not to smoke." We kept all our cigarette butts in a Mason jar someplace where we'd see it often; mine was on the kitchen sink. On top, I had an appalling picture of a man who'd had radical surgery for throat cancer who was still smoking through a little hole in his neck. It was disgusting.

I had a plumber come in while I was taking the course, and he saw this thing on my sink. He stared at it for a minute, and then he said, "I've been in a lot of houses, and I've seen a lot of things, but could you please tell me what this is?" So I told him and explained about the class. He told me his girlfriend smoked and he really hated it and asked if I could get him a copy of the picture so he could give it to her. So I sent him one when I paid the bill.

At the same time that I was quitting, I lost seventeen pounds. Everyone says when you quit, you get fat as a goose. I didn't. I substituted walking for eating. I was doing a lot of healthy things to take care of myself, and I was feeling good and looking good. It was great.

RAY P.
I Finally Quit on Valentine's Day

*Ray, in his early forties, has been a hairstylist for twenty-five
years. He now owns his own unisex salon. A single parent for the
past five years, he lives with his two children, aged twenty and
seventeen. Ray has played on local baseball teams for many years.
He also coaches a girls' high school basketball team in his free
time. He found his own idiosyncratic motivation to stop.*

My smoking had a direct correlation to stress. If there
was a lot of stress, there was a lot of smoking. If there was
less stress, there was less smoking. I smoked in junior
high school, I smoked in Vietnam, and I smoked when I
was going through my divorce.

I started playing around with cigarettes in the third
grade. I quit in the ninth grade because I was interested
in sports. If you were an athlete, you didn't smoke.
(There was also an old wives' tale that smoking stunted
your growth. I don't know if it really makes you short,
but it certainly shortens your life!)

I didn't smoke again until I was in Vietnam, with all its
anxiety, boredom, tension, and the military's cheap cigarettes. You could buy cigarettes in the PX for a dime a
pack. Time really drags standing watch, and the tendency is to fall asleep, so I smoked to stay awake. I quit
again when I was discharged in 1968—the price of ciga-

rettes was so much higher than in the Army.

I started smoking in 1982 when I was going through my divorce. In fact, that was practically the first thing I did. It was a Sunday morning, I got in the truck, went out and bought a pack of cigarettes, and smoked. Smoking has always been a crutch for me in times of stress. I started and quit several times before I finally quit in 1988.

I never smoked in front of the girls on the basketball team I coach. I felt funny about smoking in front of them. They were athletes, and I didn't want to set them a bad example. I made sure I never smoked around them because it made me feel like a hypocrite. As a matter of fact, they never knew I smoked until after they graduated and came back to visit me. Then I would light up, and they would look startled and say, "I didn't know you smoked."

I finally quit on Valentine's Day, 1988. It was very symbolic. There are lots of heart problems in my family. My mother had open-heart surgery, my father had heart trouble, I have three brothers with high blood pressure—all the indicators are there for me to have heart problems, too. I began to think seriously about the health hazards of smoking; I don't want to screw myself up. I want to eliminate one of the risk factors. I've never done drugs in my life, but my eating habits are less than ideal, and I don't exercise much when I'm not coaching. I'm not going to stop abusing my body in those ways, probably, so I thought quitting smoking was the easiest step I could take in the direction of preserving my health.

My girlfriend smokes, so in 1987 we started talking about quitting and the various programs that people join to quit. I'm not much of a joiner and I'm not a very good follower; I like to do things my own way. I find my own idiosyncratic motivations. I understand that it is very *in* for yuppies to join programs and support groups, but I didn't want to be like a yuppie. I run away from anything like that, so I used my *machismo.* I'm Mexican American, so I turned to my Latin heritage and told myself that if I smoked I was less than manly, and that a real man could do it on his own. I didn't want to join a group, like some yuppie; I could do it myself. And I did.

Quitting smoking is exactly like being in an athletic competition. The idea that you can do it starts kicking around in your head. You start telling yourself, "This is bullshit. I don't need this." You start little by little psyching yourself up. Slowly you get your thoughts together until you know what you're going to do. When the right day comes, you wake up one morning and say, "Today is the day." That's what I did on Valentine's Day, 1988. I had smoked over a pack of cigarettes a day off and on for more than thirty years.

I find I eat more now, not because I'm hungry, but for something to do. In the hairstyling business, if you're not busy, you're bored. You sit around a lot. I can do some bookkeeping, but it's still just sitting. I miss having something to do with my hands the way I did when I was smoking.

So far there hasn't been any problem, but the idea

keeps nagging me that I quit for five years once before. I liken myself to an alcoholic: I always have to be aware of the problem.

ERIC W.
An Afternoon in Jail

Eric W., now in his late forties, designs communications systems intended to survive under conditions of extreme stress, such as nuclear attack. He describes his job as "tap-dancing on quicksand." He is a serious photographer as well, with subjects ranging from vintage cars to African wildlife.

Here's the scenario. I'm thirty-five years old, and I've made this deal with myself that if I don't have to spend the night in jail I'll quit smoking. My wife arrives with the bail about ninety seconds before they close down releases for the day. Now I'm honor bound to quit, but I've got to deal with the oral gratification issue, so I fixate on Tootsie-Pops, my favorite childhood lollipop. I buy Tootsie-Pops by the bagful. My briefcase is full of Tootsie-Pops. I've got Tootsie-Pops in both pockets of my suit jacket, and I sit in meetings with the Pentagon's top brass wondering what flavors I've got left.

When I can't stand it any longer, I pull out a Tootsie-Pop, unwrap it, and start sucking. You want to bring a meeting to an abrupt halt? You want to change the subject? You want the top brass to hang on your every word? Whip out a Tootsie-Pop in a high-level Pentagon or CIA meeting. Works every time.

But let's begin at the beginning. I started smoking twice, once when I was in high school and again a few years later. I smoked for about a year and a half before I ran away to see the world with the Navy. There were fewer people in the Navy who smoked than there had been in high school, so I quit. The peer pressure to smoke wasn't there. I'd been selected for some very sophisticated training, which meant I spent a lot of time studying, and I just didn't want to be bothered with smoking.

When I started in high school I did it because my friends smoked and because I thought it was the adult thing to do. My dad smoked Camels, so I smoked Camels. They were just wretched. They made me sick the first few times I tried it. I thought you had to prove you were tough enough to take it. I thought all men had to go through that as a dues-paying exercise.

I started again two or three years later, when I was put in an extremely high-stress position. While I was in the service I was on the Western Pacific Nuclear Emergency Team. If there was a Navy weapon that was having a problem, we went out and fixed it. That was sufficiently stressful—as in life-threatening—that I was driven back to smoking. I smoked for fifteen years, until I was thirty-five and change. I started out smoking half a pack a day and ended up smoking two and a half packs a day.

In March of 1976 the police showed up at my door on a

Sunday afternoon and arrested me for failing to pay one overdue $5 parking ticket. I had just moved and apparently the notice to pay hadn't caught up with my new address. In any case, they threw me in the back of the paddy wagon and hauled me off to jail for the afternoon.

The nicest guy in the communal cell was a Hell's Angel gang leader. The rest of the guys were *really* bad. I had some cigarettes in my pocket, so I was doling out cigarettes as a means of bribery. I told myself that if I got out of there that afternoon and didn't have to spend the night in there with those bozos I would never smoke again. I would mend my ways. The decision was made while I was sitting there looking through the bars. I hadn't even been thinking about quitting before that. There was no health issue, no peer pressure, or anything else. I walked out of there without a single cigarette left, and from that moment to this I've never smoked again.

In the three or four hours that I was in jail, Carolyn, my wife, was running around to five different grocery stores, none of which would cash a check for more than $20, to raise the $100 bail. That was back before automated teller machines. She arrived at the jail seconds before they closed down releases for the day. I was down to my last cigarette.

I had a tough time with the withdrawal. The first week was relatively easy because I was on a motivational roll, but then I started to feel the physical craving for a cigarette. I realized I was going to have to deal with the oral gratification issue. I went through bag after bag of Tootsie-Pops. I ate those things constantly. It was the only thing that kept me going. I would reach into my suit coat pocket and feel five or six Tootsie-Pops and wonder what flavors I had left. I would take one out, carefully unwrap it, and then somebody would ask what I was doing. That went on for the better part of a year. I missed the security and reassurance of a cigarette, especially in situations where I had to think fast. Over the years I've learned to tap-dance on quicksand.

There wasn't a lot of support for quitting. Most people wanted to know why, and I didn't have any compelling reason like my doctor told me I'd die if I didn't. I had never questioned the habit at all. More of the people I knew smoked than didn't, so the pressure was to smoke rather than otherwise. That was the norm. The reaction most people had to the announcement that I'd quit smoking was, "What the hell did you do that for?"

The real crisis was in the 90-day to 120-day period after I quit. The frequency with which I wanted a cigarette began to spread out, but the intensity with which I wanted that cigarette got worse and worse and worse. There were times when I really considered that I wasn't going to make it. But there was no backsliding. At no time during that crunch did I ever pick one up.

I went through years and years of watching somebody else go through the ritual after a meal or a drink and living that ritual vicariously. I came close to slipping a few times, less because I wanted the nicotine than because I missed the ritual.

When the desire was greatest, I told myself that I'd never been able to deny myself anything that gave me pleasure, and this was one time I was going to do it. It was a self-test, a good cause, and a good opportunity to see if I could do it. I didn't want to let myself down.

BECKI C.
I Don't Want to Be an Addict!

Becki C., manager of a word-processing business, transcribed the interviews in this book. As she read the stories, she began to think about her own smoking habit. By the time she had finished twenty of the interviews, she was able to quit.

As I listened to the tapes of these ex-smokers, I was struck by how *addictive* nicotine is. I had smoked for more than twenty-five years and had tried quitting, just like a lot of these people, over and over again. The fact that nicotine is a drug really disturbed me. The realization that *I* was an addict was what did it for me. I had worked for years with the Pathway Drug Abuse Council and had put together drug abuse seminars. It was very upsetting to think of myself as being one of the people that I had been trying to help before. It really bothered me to recognize that I was doing something I had no control over. I don't like being in a situation where I'm not in control of myself.

It wasn't even easy for me to get started smoking. I remember standing in front of the bathroom mirror when I was fifteen or sixteen to see what I looked like smoking and watching myself turn green. I didn't smoke much then—maybe a pack a month, mostly what I could cadge from the people I babysat for. Oddly enough, most of the people for whom I babysat were physicians, and most of them smoked. They usually had cigarettes lying around the house, so after the kids were in bed and my homework was finished, I'd practice smoking.

I had smoked for almost twenty years before I tried to quit for the first time. That was in 1979. My husband at that time—a physician, by the way—was a very heavy smoker. He couldn't sit through a movie without getting up to have a cigarette. He couldn't even sleep through the night without waking up for a smoke. He went to Smokenders and quit, just like that! I figured, "If *he* can do it, I'll have no trouble at all." I went to Smokenders and paid the whole amount the first night, I was so sure I'd quit successfully. I was one of three in a class of more than sixty who didn't quit. The other two had quit by the last follow-up class I went to. Me, the one who came in bursting with confidence, sure it was going to be a snap, I didn't.

I had just bought a new BMW when I started Smokenders, so I made a rule that nobody could smoke in my new car, including me. I stuck to that rule for about four years. That was the beginning of my *selective* non-smoking.

Three years ago I had the entire interior of the house repainted and new drapes hung, so I made a rule of no smoking in the house. That one went by the wayside a little sooner. I started cheating and smoking in the bathroom when winter came, because it got awfully cold and wet going outside to smoke.

Two years ago I tried quitting again. I gained thirty pounds. I went back to smoking but managed to keep it down to a pack a day for the last two years. I wanted very badly to quit, but I was afraid of gaining more weight.

Two months ago I quit again. I'd read all these interviews I was transcribing, and I realized how addictive nicotine is. No wonder it's been hard to quit. I haven't been as tense and crabby this time. As long as I'm busy and there are things to do, it really doesn't bother me. I do have to stay away from alcohol; it lowers my defenses and makes it much harder to resist smoking. I feel I'm doing well. I want this to be the last time I quit. I don't want to be an *addict.*

JOHN A.
I Saw What Could Happen

John A. is a doctoral candidate in clinical psychology and a supervisor at a clinic that specializes in rehabilitating people who have suffered brain injuries. He also does group and individual therapy and psychological testing at a state prison, where he works as an intern. He is twenty-seven years old.

Two things made me decide to quit smoking. One was that I had been experiencing some respiratory congestion and headaches from smoking. I knew smoking was bad for me and I knew I needed to come to terms with the habit. The other, that hit very close to home, is that a good friend, a neighbor who's only sixty-three, is dying of emphysema. He's in a great deal of pain and can only walk a few steps without being out of breath. He was a heavy smoker for fifty years. He talked to me about how wise it is to stop smoking now and not risk what he is suffering in the future.

That had a big impact on me because, like me, he started smoking when he was young. I saw with my own eyes what can happen from prolonged smoking. I know him well, and he's dying slowly in a lot of pain.

I started smoking when I was eleven or twelve, in the sixth grade. It was just something to do with the neighborhood kids, not a habit, but still I smoked five or six cigarettes a week until my last year in high school. Then I quit for a year and started smoking again in college. I smoked anywhere from a couple of packs a week to half a pack a day for more than ten years, and I always smoked strong, unfiltered cigarettes, like Camels.

I'd been having headaches and nasal congestion for two years, and that disturbed me. I've always been very athletic, and I noticed I was losing my wind. It's important to me to be in good shape physically, not necessarily to compete in sports, but just to be generally fit. I knew it was because of smoking, so I decided to improve my health and do away with the silly habit.

I had tried to quit before; most smokers have! I've made many attempts over the years to stop. They all succeeded for a few months. Then I'd start again, because I was feeling stressed, or I was in a bar with a friend who was smoking.

This time I had a kind of internal dialogue with myself. I realized that the time had come to use my willpower, so I said to myself, "That's it. I'm quitting cold turkey." And that's what I did.

The first couple of weeks were very difficult. It's not easy to break a habit of ten years' duration. But once I decided that was what I was going to do, it wasn't so hard. I was in a lot of situations where I was tempted, but I didn't follow through with the temptation.

It would make sense to say that all my training in psychology helped me, but I don't think it did. I wish all that learning and education made a bigger difference, but I honestly think it was my own determination that helped me to quit for good. When I feel confident that I'm making the right decision, I have the willpower to do what I need to do.

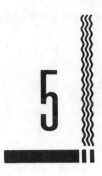

THE LESSONS OF
EXPERIENCE

THE MOMENT OF DECISION

For everyone there seems to be a moment that is right for making a major decision, for making a significant change of behavior. This is true in all kinds of addictions, where several attempts to quit are common before achieving success.

The moment of decision that leads to successful quitting is like the release of a tightly wound spring. Many people remember the day, and even the hour of their decision. Some decisions seem born of the events of a moment, as when Don C. (p. 82), suffering a serious heart attack, heard the hospital staff asking if there was a priest who could administer the last rites, or when Louise G. (p. 114) experienced an ambulance trip after

224

she blacked out, fell, and hit her head.

Some decisions to quit appear impulsive but are, in fact, often preceded by a long period of thought, emotional preparation, and unsuccessful attempts to stop smoking. The moment of decision may come as a shock—for example, the desperation, emptiness, and loneliness felt by Arlene H. (p. 206) in the few days after her husband walked out on their twenty-third wedding anniversary, never to return. Arlene's story demonstrates how extraordinary external stress can lead to the decision to quit smoking. Arlene had thought about quitting for ten years before that moment.

Other people's decisions to quit appear to be purely spur-of-the-moment. Eric W. (p. 215) was anxious not to spend the night in jail with a gang of ugly-tempered cellmates and gave away his cigarettes, one by one, as bribes. Peering through the bars, he promised himself that if he was sprung before lock-down that evening he would quit smoking.

THE POWER OF INCENTIVES

Some quitters came up with incentives for stopping that were more appealing than continuing to smoke.

Our most expensive example occurs in Mike B.'s story (p. 154), when his wife agreed to the purchase of a new Mercedes Benz, *if* he never smoked in the car. Mike took the bait and decided to quit smoking the day they drove off on their three-week cross-country trip surrounded by brand-new upholstery and its "new car smell."

Good incentives can help overcome some of the obsta-
cles to the final decision to quit smoking. There is another new-car story buried in the pre-quitting history of
Betsey W. After her husband bought her an expensive
new car, to keep it smelling fresh and new, she dis-
sociated her smoking habit from one part of her life:
driving her car (p. 177). She did not stop smoking completely for a year, but this was an important part of the
incubation process.

The potential health damage of cigarettes is the deci-
sive factor in quitting for many people. Fear is often
aroused when something happens to the smoker personally—such as a heart attack or a physical abnormality
discovered during a medical examination—or by seeing friends or family suffering from a painful, disabling,
smoking-related disease. Sometimes fear for one's
health is aroused by news items in newspapers, articles in
magazines, or radio and television programs and advertising.

Celeste Holm, the actress and singer, was afraid that
she would lose her voice, which was essential to her career, unless she stopped smoking (p. 159). All the symptoms of a small problem that could eventually threaten
her livelihood were there in Las Vegas, a place where her
nightclub act and her career depended on her singing.
Louise G. wanted to avoid fainting and falling again and
hurting herself even more seriously than she had the first
time. Fear of not being able to be physically active and
symptoms such as shortness of breath, developing a

cough, or having chest pain when they breathed deeply led several people to quit smoking.

And a healthy vanity played a part in the decision for those who dreaded the smoker's wrinkles, the dry skin, the pallor, the yellowed teeth, the tobacco-stained fingers, and the smell of stale tobacco in their hair and clothes.

Behavior changes can take place when thinking changes, and many people found the courage and strength to stop by associating powerful images, both positive and negative, with smoking.

A good positive image is to imagine yourself as a non-smoker. Visualize yourself with smoother skin, healthier color, and whiter teeth, able to breathe deeply without pain or wake up in the morning without coughing, able to taste and smell again. Think of the smell of flowers, clean mountain or sea air, and the taste of your favorite foods. Imagine yourself achieving new levels of accomplishment for whatever physical activities you do— whether it's walking up stairs without getting winded, hiking farther, running faster, or playing tennis better.

Negative or depressing images are often created by accidental events, but their impact is tremendous on the minds of smokers who have been considering quitting. Joni L. responded to the American Cancer Society television ad in which William Talman, dying of lung cancer, pleaded with the audience not to smoke (p. 90). Talman reminded Joni of her father, who had smoked and died of cancer. Joni said, "I thought about it for a couple of weeks. I could not shake the memory of that man, that wonderful actor. His face was constantly before me, even while I was at work." Joni was haunted by the image of the dying actor, coupled with her fears of the health hazards of smoking after losing both parents to cancer. The combination of the two images helped her quit.

Leslie M.'s experience also bears out the power of negative images as probably the single most effective motivation for her decision to quit was the face of a woman (p. 126). Leslie described the woman, whom she much admired: "Her skin is wrinkled and gray and her gums and teeth are yellowish, like dog's teeth." Leslie, a writer, was surrounded by talented, creative, intellectual women and men who smoked constantly. Leslie saw herself beginning to look like some of her friends and decided to quit smoking.

Amanda M. admired the actor who played Latka on the television series "Taxi," a man only a year older than she was. When she learned that the actor had died of lung cancer, she said: "Oh, God, this is horrible. He is only a little bit older, and he died of this weird cancer" (p. 52). This image was coupled with a statistic she had read that said that there is a certain number of cigarettes that can be smoked before the next one might cause serious disease. Every time she smoked, she coupled the thought of that statistic with the image of Latka, and the combination pushed her toward her decision.

Many images came from something that was read or seen: A picture of a man who had only tubes where his throat had been, still smoking, is known to have influenced many people in the 1970s.

Some images are drawn from experiences closer to home. James V.'s uncle lived in his house for the last few months of his life, and the pain he suffered from lung cancer made James determined to quit smoking (p. 63). A neighbor of whom he was very fond and who was suffering from emphysema warned John A. of the dangers of smoking, and John heeded his warning (p. 221). He could see himself ending up like his sad, shuffling neighbor if he kept smoking. Allen S. described eloquently the devastating impact of visiting a friend who had had a heart attack (p. 163): "It was awful. His wife was waiting in the hallway [of the hospital] wringing her hands. He was trying to put up a good front for his kids and me. He hadn't shaved in a while, he didn't have much strength, and he was lying there in a private room in a little hospital. I thought, 'My God, this is awful.' It was awful for him and it was awful for everybody around him."

Effective negative images need not be so direct. David Goerlitz, the Winston Man, realized that he was helping cigarette companies recruit new young smokers by symbolizing a good-looking, healthy, active young man—the kind of person kids want to be—in Winston's advertising (p. 69). Seeing children twelve to thirteen years of age buying cigarettes triggered the guilt that led to his decision to quit smoking *and* quit modeling for the Winston commercials.

CREATING YOUR OWN POWERFUL IMAGES

Your own personal images will help you quit smoking. And you can create them without having a heart attack, or watching a neighbor die of emphysema, by using a combination of positive and negative images.

As you are working toward the decision to quit and strengthening your motivation, imagine yourself achieving a new level of physical fitness. Visualize how much better your clothes, car, and house would smell if they were free of stale smoke.

Then create negative images, such as a lung full of tar. If a clear image doesn't come to you, hold a sponge in your hand and pour molasses over it. Then squeeze out the sponge, and think of it as your lung with the tars that have accumulated from years of smoking oozing out. This image was used in a public service advertisement in Australia and was extremely effective. It was identified by thousands of people as having a major impact on their decision to quit.

Imagine a person dying of emphysema, gaunt, with a thin, haggard face, a grayish pallor, walking with halting steps and scarcely able to breathe. People with emphysema cannot take a deep breath—every breath is shallow—and doctors can recognize people with early emphysema from twenty feet away by the way they breathe—or, more accurately, don't breathe. Call up that image as part of your decision-making process.

In addition to lung-related problems, cigarettes cause thick, fatty cholesterol deposits to develop in the coronary arteries, the arteries that bring blood to the heart muscle. Most people are more afraid of contracting cancer of the lung than they are of a heart attack, but the fact is, cigarettes cause more heart attacks than they do lung cancer. Smokers are known to have two to four times more coronary attacks than non-smokers.

Imagine the inside of a coronary artery. It is pink and lovely, the red blood cells are floating by, the artery is opening and closing as the blood pulses through it, and it is alive and wonderful. Then imagine what happens as a smoker continues to smoke. Thick, yellowish cholesterol sludge builds up along the sides of the artery over a ten- to twenty-year period until 60 percent of the artery is clogged. The blood has a tough time flowing through it, and a heart attack looms on the horizon.

PERSONAL TRANSFORMATION

Most people in this book, after trying to quit smoking and failing, reported achieving a different state of mind, a different level of conviction, and even a degree of inner tranquility that convinced them that *this* attempt to quit would be the last one.

Marion R. (p. 77) wrote a book about her own life in which she was "able to forgive myself for some of the things I needed to forgive myself for, pat myself on the back for some of the things that I deserved to be patted for. I made peace with some of the figures in my past, made peace with myself partially. I told myself I couldn't make peace with myself totally if I let smoking control me. . . . I woke up one morning and said, 'This is it.' I had the feeling that the monkey was off my back."

Ray P. (p. 212) challenged himself to use his Latin heritage to help him quit smoking. As he put it, it was a "macho" thing to do, because he considered it unmanly to keep smoking when he wanted to quit. It was more macho to quit cold turkey, without the support of a group or seminar, and he reinforced his decision by deciding that this was a macho, not "yuppie," way of doing it.

Elton W. came to look at quitting in a new way (p. 200). "The key thing was that I changed my attitude toward quitting entirely." He had felt like a martyr on all his previous attempts. "I would go three days without cigarettes and feel that I deserved the Congressional Medal of Honor *and* the Nobel Peace Prize." His change of attitude was precipitated by editing a book that in one section discussed why no one likes emphysema patients, including they themselves. The editing job forced him to see the health hazards of smoking in a different light.

Another rather similar personal transformation occurred during the writing of this book. After transcribing twenty interviews, Becki C. (p. 219) convinced herself that nicotine was, in fact, addicting, and she didn't want to see herself as an addict. June H.'s battles with frequent relapses and broken promises to herself ended when she

convinced herself that she had to live up to her commitment to her daughter and her daughter's friends that she
would quit when her daughter graduated from high
school (p. 119). Allen S. made many earlier attempts to
quit only "because I felt I should." But his last attempt
was different: "This time I really wanted to quit." He
made a commitment to his family two months before he
quit and used the powerful image of his friend's heart
attack and bypass operation to give him the strength to
follow through with it.

All of the people above finally took responsibility for
their habit. Once that was acknowledged, the personal
transformation became possible.

HOW TO ACHIEVE PERSONAL
TRANSFORMATION AND SELF-CONFIDENCE

If you're a heavy smoker, how can you achieve personal
transformation? Does this sound like an impossible
quest? The stories in this book show that each one of
these people did it. But you need to surmount the barrier
of negative thinking that is inside each person addicted
to smoking, a barrier that keeps you from reaching the
level of confidence where you can say, "I have stopped.
This is the last time."

This confidence gradually comes during the incubation period described on page 33 and easily recognized
in many of the stories. Recall how many of the men and

women had that inner feeling that "this is the day." With patience and awareness, you can reach the point where there is a level of inner peace and strength that says your chances are good that you can make it.

For some successful quitters that point is achieved during a calm period in their lives—when they are on vacation or when job pressures are less. For others a period of maximum stress is the time to take on the challenge of giving up smoking; quitting then becomes a distraction from the stress. Either way, you must feel certain that you are ready. You must have the confidence you can carry it through.

For some, this confidence comes as the person is solving other health problems. Succeeding at one thing gives the confidence needed to succeed in others. Success is contagious. Lesser behavioral changes can also point the way. Taking small steps, such as improving your nutrition by eating fresh fruit instead of sweets or increasing the amount of your daily exercise by walking briskly for thirty minutes at lunch, can build the confidence you need to take a big step like quitting smoking.

Many of our quitters gained confidence by realizing that they had succeeded, *at least temporarily*, in previous quit attempts. They borrowed various methods that they learned from each quit attempt—such as planning rewards during the first week or two—and then used a number of these techniques to quit once and for all. They also gave up blaming themselves for the failure of previous attempts, concentrating on the aspects that were successful instead of saying, "I'll *never* be able to quit."

WHAT ABOUT FRIENDS AND RELATIVES?

Many non-smoking spouses have waited for years for their partners to quit. Remember Steve G.? He told us: "A fact which I now think is marvelous is that she [his wife] could live with a smoker for four years, because now [as a non-smoker] I am so intolerant of it myself. Just the smell, the ashtrays, and everything else." Steve looked back and realized how much his wife had put up with.

Smokers need to accept the pressure to stop smoking from friends and relatives in the loving spirit with which it is intended—these people want you to live a longer, healthier life. Friends and family should be careful to express their feelings in a gentle and loving way without resorting to nagging. At the same time they should recognize that the response of smokers may well be to reject that advice, sometimes for years, before they're ready to stop smoking.

Bob L.'s story (p. 111) is an interesting reversal, indicating true generosity of spirit. Bob was perfectly content to continue smoking but stopped because his wife wanted to quit, and he realized it would be easier for her if he stopped smoking at the same time. June H. broke innumerable promises to herself to quit smoking, but when she kept her promise to her daughter to quit the day she was graduated from high school she was successful. Commitments can feel stronger if you say them aloud, or better yet write them down and have a friend or relative sign your statement that you intend to quit.

Sometimes, of course, friends can hamper your efforts: When Eric W.'s friends realized that he had quit smoking, they said, "What in the hell did you do that for?" It was up to Eric to rise above their reactions to his new resolve. Social pressure to smoke is still significant. Preparing yourself for possible negative reactions is as important as asking your friends and family to support you in your effort to quit.

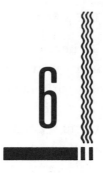

LIFE AFTER SMOKING

THE FIRST WEEK

According to all of our ex-smokers, the first week was the hardest. Eric W. was the sole exception. In Eric's case, he was on a "motivational roll" the first week. His trouble started later, when he felt the need for oral gratification as a delayed reaction. In all the stories there is a common theme of a need to keep hands busy by playing with rubber bands, fiddling with glasses, or shredding paper cups; a need for oral gratification that was satisfied by eating Tootsie-Pops, munching celery or carrot sticks, and even sucking orange juice from a baby bottle. Some people learned to wait out the urge to smoke by taking a brief, brisk walk or closing the eyes and giving a pep talk on how important it is not to have the first cigarette.

237

Leslie M.'s letters to her friend give a day-to-day history of what happened during the first week. "Today marks exactly one week without a cigarette, and though it's a lot better than it was the first three days, I am still missing cigs a lot. The first three days were hell. I was feeling crazy, mean, restless, and had terrific nightmares in which I was smoking like crazy. When I woke up, my chest hurt as if I had been chain-smoking; my throat was sore and I felt positively battered. The next few nights, I couldn't sleep at all. I got up and wandered around the house in the dark sucking on toothpicks and wanting a cigarette so badly I thought I'd get dressed and go out to an all-night store. But I held out. I inspect my face every day now to find the changes—the slow but wonderful changes in my skin and hair. . . . In order to keep myself from wanting cigs, I've taken endless bike rides and am enjoying the way my lungs feel better and cleaner every day. I can't believe how much more breath I have. . . . Probably my single greatest benefit in quitting smoking is what I can smell now—since I am a person who responds so much to smell. . . . There's something very sensuous about not smoking. I want to touch everyone, get close, smell skin. I want to put my nose against heads and shoulders and arms. I smell my own skin, my hands and wrists and breasts. It's quite wonderful and sexy. I feel sort of sexually charged by it all and wonder if I haven't been missing out on something all of these years."

Leslie gives us a window through which we see some of the suffering of ex-smokers, particularly those who had smoked more than a pack and a half a day. She tells us of the value of distractions—in her case, the extensive cycling and the joy of regaining her sense of smell, which enhanced the sense of her own sexuality. She speaks of the exhilaration of feeling fit and healthy, breathing deeply, and seeing tone and color in her face.

John G., another heavily addicted smoker, reports his feeling of triumph at getting through the first week: "I had a great sense of victory." His advice to smokers is to distract themselves. "Go to four movies a week, take up needlepoint. Just don't think about what a poor, unloved child you are because you've quit smoking." He is right about the self-pity, incidentally, a realization that probably led to his final successful attempt to quit.

Among our stories the choice of distractions is varied. More than one person chose walking; one man has a dish of rubber bands or a coin ready so that when he is in meetings he can act like Captain Queeg in *The Caine Mutiny*. Another tells us about carrot and celery sticks, and still another recommends Tootsie-Pops. Steve G. dealt with oral gratification in the most direct possible way, sucking orange juice from a baby bottle while he watched television for a few weeks after he stopped smoking.

In waiting for the urge to smoke to go away, there are some good tips from Patrick Reynolds (p. 95): "Take it easy, the desire will be gone in five minutes, so just wait it out. I make a conscious decision not to have a cigarette at that tempting moment. I haven't smoked for four years, and now those moments occur much less often." Betsey W. found that after several minutes the urge for a cigarette would go away. Michael G. found that a computer keyboard kept his hands busy when he wanted to reach for a smoke. In a rather unusual method of quelling the urge to smoke, Joni L. allowed herself to sleep for three days. After that the urge to smoke was gone.

Elton W.'s story shows the power of imagining yourself in a new role, or practicing a new role. He found the long trip over the bridge that carries commuters from their hideaways to their workdays in a big city a marvelous opportunity to practice being the non-smoker he wanted to be. He pretended in the car that he was a "squeaky clean purist who would be shocked and offended by smoking." He imagined another person offering a cigarette to him. He would say, over and over again when this person offered a cigarette, "No, thanks, I don't smoke." "God knows what the other commuters thought of me smiling, nodding pleasantly, and obviously talking to myself every morning and evening." In psychologists' jargon this is called *cognitive restructuring*, which is the action of practicing a new behavior. It is a form of playacting in which you take the role of the person you wish to become. Acting and practicing this role makes it easier to do in real life.

Change of environment is another way to deal with the early days after quitting. Mike B. was away from home and work for three weeks, touring the country in a new car. Another of our interviewees did the same, quitting while he was on vacation with his family.

Counteracting some of the physical cravings of the body by using nicotine gum is another way to prevent relapse in the first weeks after quitting. Neil B. (p. 139) found the use of nicotine gum helpful. Usually the gum should be used for a few months, always under a physician's careful supervision, tapering the dose down to zero in the last few weeks. Some people purposely allow themselves a moderate use of alcohol and coffee and eat whatever they want during the first week in order to avoid feeling deprived and sorry for themselves. The Alcoholics Anonymous principle of "one day at a time" can help you to get through the first week. Steve G. says, "I quit one day at a time."

You should expect some discomfort during the first week if you were a heavy smoker. The stories provide graphic descriptions, but fortunately these feelings do not last too long. The time for these feelings to totally disappear varies from person to person. For some people they may last as long as two or three weeks.

Use distractions to allay the discomfort and be ingenious in finding distractions that best suit you. Cultivate activities with your hands; munch on celery, carrots, or fruit; walk, swim, or play tennis. Visualize images of peaceful tranquility and glowing good health. Make changes in your world. Don't try to give up coffee, sugar, and alcohol at the same time you quit smoking. Be gentle with yourself. Don't punish yourself by giving up everything you like just because you're quitting smoking. Not smoking is a step in the direction of a longer, healthier life, not a punishment.

When the urge to smoke strikes, wait it out. After a minute or two the urge goes away. Use your favorite distractions during that time. Keep in mind that each day that passes reduces the amount of nicotine in your body and thus reduces the level of physical dependence as well.

Choose a time to quit when you can make a change in your environment and get away. Even a long weekend away may make it a bit easier to get through the first week of non-smoking. A longer trip is even better. In changing environments, you're probably reducing stress, and that's a bonus in itself.

THE LONG TERM

Some of the methods that are helpful in the first week are good for the long term, too. Although physical addiction to nicotine fades away in a few weeks, people do remain vulnerable to relapse, perhaps for the rest of their lives. The likelihood that relapse will occur diminishes monthly to the point where after a few years it is quite unlikely. There are a few examples of people who went back to smoking after as long as seven years, however, and Dick W. (p. 15) began again after fifteen years. The trick is never to think that one cigarette won't make any difference; it does. Steve G. (p. 168) had been off cigarettes for six months and had gained some weight. This led him to toy with the idea of doing a little bit of smoking. "When I started smoking again I did it by taking just one drag on a cigarette, and that was it—I was off to the races. In view of my experiences in A.A. where one drink starts you drinking again, I should have realized that one cigarette was going to take me back down the same road." Again, as soon as the urge comes, realize that it will go away in a few minutes. If you need help, try visualization techniques. Imagine all the benefits of being a non-smoker in concrete detail.

Don't be deluded, as Mike B. was, by the notion that smoking cigars is not as addictive. Thinking he could smoke just one or two a day, in five months he was up to twelve cigars a day. He realized then that he "couldn't ever touch tobacco in any form."

A good long-term coping skill is to be constantly aware of the kinds of situations that can cause slips or relapses: the stress of divorce, a change of job, unemployment, unexpected stress, and, all too often, too much to drink. Even having one drink cuts down on inhibitions and this—especially in the first few months after quitting— may lead you to think, "Oh, what the hell; just one cigarette won't hurt me." In Alcoholics Anonymous this is what is called "stinkin' thinkin,'" and it's the kind of distorted thinking alcohol causes. Sidestepping a drink is an example of discretion being the better part of valor, at least until you feel completely secure in your status as a non-smoker.

The desire for a cigarette may be especially intense in particular, familiar situations. Even such a strong anti-smoking advocate as Patrick Reynolds occasionally feels the desire for a cigarette after a meal. "The hardest times for me even now are when I am relaxed, say, on vacation at a friend's estate. I have had a beautiful meal, we are having an espresso, a friend lights up a cigarette, and I really, *really* want one. It is as though everything is perfect except that one thing is missing: *my* cigarette."

Make a list of the activities or circumstances you associate with smoking, such as turning on the ignition of your car, having a cup of coffee, or the quiet period after solving a difficult problem. The chance meeting of an old friend who invites you to have a drink and offers you a cigarette may bring back memories of all the times you talked and drank and smoked. Then make a second list of all the positive things about *not* smoking. Make a third list of all the negative aspects of smoking. Carry your lists around with you, and when a tempting situation arises, review your second and third lists to reinforce your determination not to smoke ever again.

MAKING USE OF MENTAL IMAGES

To sidestep the temptation to smoke, use *positive images*: freedom from the foul smell of stale tobacco smoke, freedom from all the paraphernalia of smoking, freedom from the dirty ashtrays filled with cigarette butts, freedom from the coughing and irritated throat of the smoking years, freedom from the headaches, the renewed ability to smell and taste, and your new sense of physical fitness. Visualize your clean, healthy lungs and arteries, and remember that you are now far less likely to suffer the pain and disability of heart and lung disease. Think of yourself as an intelligent person who is no longer addicted to tobacco smoke.

If you need more help to bolster your decision not to smoke, project *negative images.* Think of dying of emphysema or heart disease, or a friend's bypass surgery. Fight the urge to smoke with a mental counterattack. Make it visual. Imagine the face of an emphysema patient with his larynx removed still smoking, and imagine yourself like that.

Reverse imagery works. Remember Leslie M. and her description of a woman smoker's face? "She's a great lady, feisty, older, smart—but her face is positively an example of the smoker's face they show you in those scare tactic programs. It's true that smoking ages the skin in a way nothing else does. Women who have smoked for a long time begin to look like ashtrays themselves. This woman is a prime example. Her skin is wrinkled and gray, and her gums and teeth are yellowish like dog teeth. If you look hard, you see that this woman is neither very old nor naturally very ugly. She also has that thinning, limp smoker's hair and yellowish fingers. I was so frightened of becoming like that that I was motivated to quit."

IF A SLIP OCCURS

All the stories in this book point out that one cigarette, even after years without smoking, can cause a relapse that can lead to a full-fledged habit again. Don't believe that after years of non-smoking you can smoke *just* one cigarette on a special occasion and never touch a cigarette again, or that you can smoke a cigarette once a month and not become addicted again.

If you slip and smoke a cigarette, stop immediately. Do not think that just because you have smoked one you might as well smoke another, or that since one doesn't seem to have caused any terrible harm you can finish the pack and then stop.

While you should try to avoid a slip at any cost, you must also not despair if you slip after not smoking for a while. Don't flog yourself with self-criticism, don't say, "I don't have any willpower. I am no good. What the hell, I might as well smoke again." Be positive. Think, "All that time, and only one cigarette. That's pretty good!" Remember how good and clean it felt when you weren't smoking. Call up the smell of stale smoke on your clothes and car, the awful images of clogged arteries, the gasping breathing of emphysema patients, and the horrors of lung cancer.

And stop right there, with that one cigarette.

ON THE RIGHT PATH

The fact that you are reading this book suggests that you are at least thinking of giving up smoking. If you have already quit, it suggests you want to learn how to avoid starting again. Consider that the reading of this book, even if it was given to you by a friend, is a positive move in the right direction. Use the ideas you find in the stories and picture yourself as a non-smoker, using the methods that work best for you.

Move toward the decision to quit thoughtfully. Let it incubate. Learn more about smoking and what it does. Learn more about quitting and what it can do for you. Read again the interviews that most closely parallel your smoking patterns and habits. Move toward building your confidence, conviction, and commitment to quit.

As noted earlier, there is a right time to quit. It is usually a period of relative tranquility in your life, even if only for a week or two. It could be at the beginning of a vacation or when there are no major changes coming up in your work or personal life.

But the right time could be a stressful time, a time when you might feel that since everything else is going wrong quitting smoking is one good thing you could do for yourself. Pick the time that feels right for you.

ANALYZE YOUR DEGREE OF ADDICTION

It is helpful to know whether or not you are a heavily addicted smoker and whether or not some extra help is needed to quit successfully. Determine your degree of addiction by using this simplified scoring system:

1. **Do you smoke more than:**
   2 packs a day? Give yourself 6 points.
   25 cigarettes a day? Give yourself 4 points.
   **Between 10 and 20 cigarettes a day? Give yourself
     1 point.**

2. **Do you continue smoking even if you have a cold?
   If yes, add 4 points.**

3. **When do you have your first cigarette of the day?
   Before breakfast = 4 points.
   After breakfast = 2 points.
   After lunch = 1 point.**

Heavily addicted: score greater than 11
Intermediate: 4 to 11
Light: less than 3

If you scored higher than 11 points, you are heavily addicted. It is highly likely that you have inherited a tendency to respond to nicotine differently from those who are able to smoke less than a pack a day. Even though science has not found the answer as to why nicotine affects different people in different ways, we know that quitting is more difficult for people who are heavily addicted. If you are in this category, you might consider using nicotine chewing gum, prescribed by your doctor, when you quit. Use nicotine chewing gum if you have failed once or twice before. Neil B. and his wife used it for two months in their last, and successful, attempt to quit smoking. Heavily addicted smokers must recognize the fact of addiction and be especially kind to themselves when they quit.

Moderate smokers (scores between 4 and 11) need to take their efforts to quit seriously and use whatever techniques will help them stay away from cigarettes. Use the power of mental images (p. 230) in both a positive and a negative way.

Lightly addicted smokers (scores of 3 or less) should be able to quit without drugs like nicotine gum.

FUTURE DEVELOPMENTS:
DRUGS AND PROGRAMS FOR THOSE
WHO WANT TO BREAK THE HABIT

Nicotine gum is an example of a prescription drug that helps not only in quitting but also in preventing relapse in the first few months after quitting. Many people object to replacing the nicotine from cigarettes with nicotine from chewing gum. Yet for a month or two for heavily addicted people, it may be kindest to have something that allows you to decrease the psychological addiction before you go cold turkey on zero nicotine.

New drugs that could help the heavily addicted smoker are currently being tested. These drugs must be used under careful medical supervision. Clonidine, previously used to lower blood pressure, is now under study, in combination with nicotine-containing chewing gum, as an aid to heavily addicted people who have failed many previous quit attempts. Recently, a few anti-depressant drugs have shown some benefit, and nicotine-containing skin patches will soon be available. Any drug has to be used with great caution to avoid substituting one addiction for another.

Scientists and physicians who have worked with these drugs are unanimous in emphasizing that confidence-building and coping skills are the basic foundation of quitting smoking successfully. Intervention with powerful drugs should be undertaken only to decrease initial stress and improve the smoker's chances of staying away from cigarettes. Drugs should be as temporary as crutches for a sprained ankle.

All around the United States people have increased their awareness of the dangers of smoking. Businesses are sponsoring programs that help people to quit. The regulations against secondhand smoke have restricted places where smokers can smoke: Motivation for work sites includes the fact that employee productivity lost to smoking is a serious consideration in the short term, and the cost of medical benefits coverage is a significant capital expenditure in the long term.

Research shows that young people may never start smoking if they are given short courses in how to resist peer pressure. These studies give hope that young people can sidestep smoking in the early teen years, when most people become addicted. Of course, the best way to reduce the appeal smoking has for kids who want to be perceived as grown-up is to make smoking something *real grown-ups don't do.*

HELP OTHERS WHO STILL SMOKE

Giving this book to a friend or relative is a good first step. If you are an ex-smoker who used this book in your decision to quit, your example is a strong statement in itself: Don't underestimate this.

You can do more: Learn how to become a helpful supporter. Nagging doesn't help; quiet encouragement does. Let people know that you will support them if they decide to stop. This is often enough to give smokers who are thinking about quitting the extra motivation they need to do it. You can also become more active (and persistent) if you sense a green light exists.

You can act as a hotline for telephone support or be a jogging or walking partner during the first few weeks of quitting. You can also sign a contract that states your support in a general way.

This book is based on the premise that the inspiration of ex-smokers and their own stories, told in their own way, is the best way to be inspired and to learn how to quit or to stay off if you have already quit. The drama of the life of an ex-smoker is much more intriguing than any scientific lecture.